The ESC Handbook of Cardiovascular Rehabilitation

T0202404

EUROPEAN SOCIETY OF CARDIOLOGY PUBLICATIONS

FORTHCOMING

The ESC Handbook of Cardiovascular Rehabilitation

Editors

Ana Abreu
Cardiovascular Rehabilitation Centre of CHULN and FMUL,
Department of Cardiology, Hospital Santa Maria, CHULN, Lisbon
Faculty of Medicine of the University of Lisbon (FMUL),
Lisbon, Portugal

Jean-Paul Schmid
Department of Cardiology, Clinic Barmelweid, Barmelweid,
Switzerland

Massimo Francesco Piepoli
Heart Failure Unit, Cardiology, Guglielmo da Saliceto Hospital,
Piacenza, University of Parma
Institute of Life Sciences, Sant'Anna School of Advanced Studies,
Pisa, Italy

Editorial Assistant

Jorge A Ruivo
Cardiovascular Rehabilitation Centre of CHULN and FMUL,
Department of Cardiology, Hospital Santa Maria, CHULN,
Lisbon, Portugal

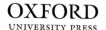

OXFORD
UNIVERSITY PRESS

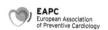

EAPC
European Association
of Preventive Cardiology

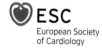

ESC
European Society
of Cardiology

OXFORD
UNIVERSITY PRESS

Great Clarendon Street, Oxford, OX2 6DP,
United Kingdom

Oxford University Press is a department of the University of Oxford.
It furthers the University's objective of excellence in research, scholarship,
and education by publishing worldwide. Oxford is a registered trade mark of
Oxford University Press in the UK and in certain other countries

Published in the United States of America by Oxford University Press
198 Madison Avenue, New York, NY 10016, United States of America

British Library Cataloguing in Publication Data

Data available

Library of Congress Control Number: 2020937824

ISBN 978-0-19-884930-8

Printed and bound by
CPI Group (UK) Ltd, Croydon, CR0 4YY

Foreword

Until recently cardiac rehabilitation has been the poor relation of cardiovascular medicine. For several years it was only performed in a few places where enthusiasts organized rehabilitation programmes. It was a long time before scientific evidence was provided which changed the way the medical community now regards cardiac rehabilitation.

Today cardiac rehabilitation has been 'rehabilitated' and is present and recommended in all the guidelines produced by the main organizations around the world. Many cardiovascular departments in a number of countries now have organized programmes of cardiac rehabilitation. However, there are still several obstacles that have to be identified in order to apply the best solutions. A fundamental obstacle is the need for appropriate education of the medical community that is potentially more involved with the use and recommendation of cardiac rehabilitation. That is where this book plays a central role. It provides comprehensive information, from basic principles to the organization of cardiac rehabilitation centres, including a detailed description of the practical aspects of developing and implementing cardiac rehabilitation in a variety of settings and populations. It is based on the recommendations of the European Association of Preventive Cardiology (EAPC) of the European Society of Cardiology (ESC), but also includes relevant information based on the extensive experience of the authors. It is the first structured comprehensive EAPC publication dealing with cardiac rehabilitation will certainly be an important milestone in the field.

This book will also make an important contribution to promoting cardiac rehabilitation (cardiovascular rehabilitation in a broader sense) on a global scale, particularly in places where there are difficulties in developing appropriate rehabilitation programmes, or even reluctance to do so. The World Heart Federation (WHF), as a global organization, is also engaged in promoting good practice around the world and identifies itself with projects, such as this one, coming from one of its strategic partners with an enormous potential to help in the global promotion of cardiovascular rehabilitation.

We live in a very complex world and at the time of writing this foreword we are facing the greatest challenge of our generation—the coronavirus pandemic. We will only be able to overcome this enormous challenge through the global cooperation by the medical and scientific community. Whatever the outcome of this crisis, the need for global cooperation will certainly be reinforced, and that is where projects such as this book can help to disseminate knowledge and implement programmes that can help people to live longer and better.

Congratulations to the editors, the authors, and EAPC/ESC.

Fausto J Pinto
University of Lisbon, Portugal
Past President of the ESC
President Elect of the WHF

Preface

This book is intended as a practical handbook on the implementation of rehabilitation for cardiovascular patients in clinical practice. Part of the mission of the European Association of Preventive Cardiology (EAPC), of the European Society of Cardiology (ESC), is to promote the education of healthcare professionals on this subject and this book will help to overcome many barriers.

Despite the fact that 'cardiac rehabilitation' is the most commonly used term, the editors prefer the term 'cardiovascular rehabilitation' because of its broader meaning, covering preventive measures in all cardiovascular patients. Underlying pathophysiological mechanisms and preventive interventions and strategies extend beyond the heart to the whole cardiovascular system, and to other systems too. Also, the scope of rehabilitation has grown fast and includes increasingly complex patients. More indications will surely be present in future editions.

In this respect, although the term 'cardiac rehabilitation' is often used in the book, 'cardiovascular rehabilitation' should be considered a more appropriate, inclusive, precise, and less restrictive term. The editors expect that this term will become the predominant term in the near future and therefore decided to keep it in the title of this book.

We hope you will enjoy reading this book as much as we enjoyed preparing it. Please do not hesitate to contact us with your advice, comments, and criticism, all of which will be considered for future editions.

Ana Abreu
Jean-Paul Schmid
Massimo Francesco Piepoli

Introduction

Why cardiovascular or cardiac rehabilitation?

Cardiovascular disease (CVD) prevention is defined as a coordinated set of actions, at the population level or targeted at an individual, that are aimed at eliminating or minimizing the impact of CVD and their related disabilities. Despite the significant reduction in morbidity and mortality over the past decades, CVD remains the number one cause of death in the world. More than four million people die from CVD each year in Europe, mainly due to coronary heart disease.

A lot of progress has been made in the treatment of the disease, with greater access to procedural interventions and pharmacological treatment. Nevertheless, up to one in every five patients admitted to the hospital for a myocardial infarction (MI) has a subsequent MI or stroke within the first year. Secondary prevention is crucial in reducing these recurrence rates and improving cardiovascular health in the long-term.

An important and cost-effective secondary prevention strategy is cardiac rehabilitation (CR), a multifactorial, multidisciplinary and comprehensive intervention which started in the 1960s. It has been shown to reduce mortality, hospital readmissions, and costs, and to improve exercise capacity, quality of life, and psychological well-being. CR programmes, or better-named cardiovascular rehabilitation programmes, should be well organized and meet minimal criteria to ensure optimal quality to be able to prove their merit.

The ESC prevention guidelines recommend participation in a CR programme for all hospitalized patients following an acute coronary event or revascularization, and for patients with heart failure. Even with these recommendations, CR remains under-utilized with less than 50% of patients participating in a CR programme after an acute event. CR uptake needs to be promoted and healthcare professionals should be made aware of the importance of CR and given proper guidance on how to implement the recommendations. Prevention seems more important than ever. Why should we treat a disease if we can prevent it? This handbook is part of the preventive cardiology curriculum and is the next step in the transition towards our own unique subspecialty, the Preventive Cardiologist.

Improving the quality of care

The European Association of Preventive Cardiology (EAPC) provides a comprehensive approach towards CVD prevention by incorporating it as a key aspect in every phase of life. One of the objectives is to promote excellence in education about and practice of CR, not only in the short run but throughout life. There are many ways in which the EAPC contributes to this objective. CR has a prominent place at the annual congress organized by the EAPC. New evidence is presented, new guidelines are explained, and new developments are discussed. Multiple courses on preventive cardiology and CR are organized and endorsed regularly by experts from the EAPC. In addition, educational materials and webinars are created and shared. Various decision-making tools, such as the Expert tool and HeartQoL, have been developed to support healthcare professionals in their daily practice. A patient education website has been created to offer concise and reliable information on primary and secondary prevention, including CR, to the public. Raising awareness among patients will increase adherence to therapy. The quality of care in CR centres throughout Europe is monitored and promoted through the EAPC accreditation system. Every centre that meets a set of predefined criteria, which ensure that the care delivered is up to date and of sufficient quality, can request accreditation for a minimum of three years. All of these actions have the purpose of further improving the quality of cardiovascular rehabilitation throughout Europe and support centres in all possible ways.

Why is this handbook needed?

A lot of information is available on why CR should be performed and in which types of patient. It has a permanent place in any book on secondary prevention. There are also many academic textbooks focusing on the pathophysiological aspects of exercise and rehabilitation. However, there is currently no book available that provides guidance on adequate organization of a CR centre and the management of CR patients in a comprehensive, structured, and practical manner that is consistent with the guidelines.

Because of the diversity of healthcare organizations and infrastructure in ESC member states, the information in this handbook can be tailored to your own context. For example, it answers questions on alternative models of CR (such as hospital-based versus home-based rehabilitation) and on changing technologies.

CR requires the input and expertise of a whole range of healthcare professionals, and this handbook was developed using this holistic approach. The perspective of all healthcare professionals involved is taken into account. As CR is not a 'one size fits all' solution, different patient types and the different aspects of CR are described. How do you deal with high-risk patients? What about low-risk patients? And the elderly and frail? How to deal with depression? Return to work?

A particular challenge is adherence to medication and lifestyle recommendations. This book provides a specific chapter on the factors that are important for adherence and the strategies that can be used to improve it.

This handbook is the perfect supplement to the *ESC Handbook of Preventive Cardiology* and the *ESC Textbook of Preventive Cardiology* and provides practical tools for use in everyday clinical situations, supported by science and evidence. It is the result of the contribution of and collaboration between the best experts in cardiac rehabilitation in Europe. I would like to congratulate and thank the authors for this excellent endeavour and I hope that you enjoy reading this handbook on cardiovascular rehabilitation and that it will guide you in your daily practice.

Paul Dendale
Arne Janssen

Contents

Contributors

Ana Abreu
Cardiovascular Rehabilitation Centre
of CHULN and FMUL, Department of
Cardiology, Hospital S. Maria, CHULN,
Lisbon; Faculty of Medicine of the
University of Lisbon (FMUL),
Lisbon, Portugal
Chapters 4, 14, and 15

Manuela Abreu
Department of Psychiatry, Hospital
Santa Maria, CHULN
Faculty of Medicine of University of
Lisbon, Lisbon, Portugal
Chapter 12

Marco Ambrosetti
Istituti Clinici Scientifici Maugeri,
Care and Research Institute of Pavia,
Department of Cardiac Rehabilitation,
Pavia, Italy
Chapter 17

Cindel Bonneux
Expertise Center for Digital Media,
Faculty of Sciences, Hasselt University,
Diepenbeek, Belgium
Chapter 19

Karin Coninx
Expertise Centre for Digital Media,
Faculty of Sciences, Hasselt University,
Diepenbeek, Belgium
Chapter 21

Ugo Corrà
Department of Cardiology, Istituti
Clinici Scientifici Salvatore Maugeri,
IRCCS Veruno, Veruno, Italy
Chapters 2, 5, and 9

Margaret E. Cupples
Centre for Public Health, Queen's
University, Belfast, Northern Ireland
Chapters 3 and 11

Constantinos H. Davos
Cardiovascular Research Laboratory,
Biomedical Research Foundation,
Academy of Athens, Athens, Greece
Chapters 1 and 10

Paul Dendale
Department of Cardiology, Jessa
Hospital, Hasselt, Belgium
Faculty of Medicine & Life Sciences,
Hasselt University, Hasselt, Belgium
Chapters 19 and 20

Wolfram Doehner
BCRT—Berlin Institute of Health
Centre for Regenerative Therapies,
Charité Universitätsmedizin Berlin,
Berlin, Germany
Department of Cardiology (CVK);
German Centre for Cardiovascular
Research (DZHK), Partner Site Berlin,
Charité Universitätsmedizin Berlin,
Berlin, Germany
Chapter 10

Ines Frederix
Department of Cardiology, Jessa
Hospital, Hasselt, Belgium
Faculty of Medicine & Life Sciences,
Hasselt University, Hasselt, Belgium
Faculty of Medicine & Health Sciences,
Antwerp University, Antwerp, Belgium
Antwerp University Hospital (UZA),
Antwerp, Belgium.
Chapter 19 and 20

Esteban Garcia-Porrero
Cardiologist, Complejo Asistencial
Universitario de León, Spain
Chapter 17

Martin Halle
Department of Prevention and Sports
Medicine, University Hospital 'Klinikum
rechts der Isar', Technical University
Munich, Munich, Germany
DZHK (German Center for
Cardiovascular Research), partner
site Munich Heart Alliance, Munich,
Germany
Chapter 7

Dominique Hansen
REVAL—Rehabilitation Research
Center, Faculty of Rehabilitation
Sciences, Hasselt University,
Diepenbeek, Belgium
Jessa Hospital, Heart Center Hasselt,
Hasselt, Belgium
BIOMED—Biomedical Research
Center, Faculty of Medicine and
Life Sciences, Hasselt University,
Diepenbeek, Belgium
Chapters 7 and 21

Marie Christine Iliou
Cardiac Rehabilitation and Secondary
Prevention Department, Corentin
Celton, Assistance Publique Hôpitaux
de Paris, France
Chapters 6 and 11

Miguel Mendes
Department of Cardiology, Hospital
de Santa Cruz—CHLO, Carnaxide/
Portugal
Chapter 14

Luca Moderato
Heart Failure Unit, Cardiology,
Guglielmo da Saliceto Hospital,
Piacenza, and University of Parma, Italy
Chapter 18

Catherine Monpere
Cardiac Prevention and Rehabilitation
Center Bois Gibert, Mutuelle Française
Centre Val de Loire, Tours, France
Chapter 6

Roberto Pedretti
Cardiovascular Department, IRCCS
MultiMedica, Sesto San Giovanni (MI),
Italy
Chapter 13

Massimo Francesco Piepoli
Heart Failure Unit, Cardiology,
Guglielmo da Saliceto Hospital,
Piacenza, University of Parma
Institute of Life Sciences, Sant'Anna
School of Advanced Studies,
Pisa, Italy
Chapters 3 and 18

Bernhard Rauch
Institut für Herzinfarktforschung,
Ludwigshafen, Germany
Chapter 1

Rona Reibis
Center of Rehabilitation
Research, University of
Potsdam, Germany
Cardiac Outpatient Clinic, Am Park
Sanssouci, Potsdam, Germany
Klinik am See, Rehabilitation Center
for Internal Medicine, Rüdersdorf,
Germany
Chapter 16

Martijn Scherrenberg
Department of Cardiology, Jessa
Hospital, Hasselt, Belgium
Faculty of Medicine & Life Sciences,
Hasselt University, Hasselt, Belgium
Chapter 19

Jean-Paul Schmid
Department of Cardiology, Clinic
Barmelweid, Barmelweid, Switzerland
Chapters 2, 4, 5, and 9

Contributors

xvi

Aimilia Varela
Cardiovascular Research
Laboratory, Biomedical Research
Foundation, Academy of Athens,
Athens, Greece
Chapter 10

Carlo Vigorito
Department of Translational Medical
Sciences, University of Naples
Federico II,
Naples, Italy
Chapter 15

Heinz Völler
Department of Rehabilitation Medicine,
Faculty of Health Science, University of
Potsdam, Germany
Klinik am See, Rehabilitation Center
for Internal Medicine, Rüdersdorf,
Germany
Chapter 16

Matthias Wilhelm
Department of Cardiology, Inselspital,
Bern University Hospital, University of
Bern, Switzerland
Chapter 8

Contributors

xvii

Reviewers

Ugo Corrà
Department of Cardiology, Istituti
Clinici Scientifici Salvatore Maugeri,
IRCCS Veruno, Veruno, Italy

Constantinos H. Davos
Cardiovascular Research Laboratory,
Biomedical Research Foundation,
Academy of Athens, Athens, Greece

Acknowledgements

In addition to all the authors whose expertise has enabled this book, the editors wish to acknowledge all the members (past and present) of the Secondary Prevention and Cardiac Rehabilitation who contributed to the concept of this book and, also, to the Board members of EAPC who answered enthusiastically to this project.

Many thanks to all!

Abbreviations

ACE	angiotensin-converting enzyme
ACS	acute coronary syndrome
AF	atrial fibrillation
AI	artificial intelligence
AMI	acute myocardial infarction
AT1	angiotensin II type 1
BMI	body mass index
BNP	brain natriuretic peptide
BP	blood pressure
BR	breathing rate
CABG	coronary artery bypass grafting
CAD	coronary artery disease
CANTOS	Canakinumab Anti-Inflammatory Thrombosis Outcomes Study
CBT	cognitive behavioural therapy
CCS	chronic coronary syndrome
CHF	congestive heart failure
CI	confidence interval
COPD	chronic obstructive pulmonary disease
CPET	cardiopulmonary exercise testing
CR	cardiac rehabilitation
CROS	Cardiac Rehabilitation Outcomes Study
CRT	cardiac resynchronization therapy
CV	cardiovascular
CVD	cardiovascular disease
DASH	dietary approaches to stop hypertension
DM	diabetes mellitus
EAPC	European Association of Preventive Cardiology
EB	exercise-based
ECG	electrocardiogram
EE	energy expenditure
EM	early mobilization
ESC	European Society of Cardiology

EST	exercise stress test
ET	exercise training
ETS	Essential Tool Subset
EXPERT	Exercise Prescription in Everyday Practice & Rehabilitative Training
FEV1	forced expiratory volume in 1 sec
FITT	frequency, intensity, time, type
FVC	forced vital capacity
GP	general practitioner
HADS	Hospital Anxiety Depression Scale
HBCR	hybrid cardiac rehabilitation
HDL	high-density lipoprotein
HF	heart failure
HIIT	high-intensity interval training
HR	heart rate
HRQoL	health-related quality of life
HRR	heart rate reserve
hs-CRP	high-sensitivity C-reactive protein
HTN	hypertension
ICD	implantable cardioverter–defibrillator
LDL	low-density lipoprotein
LV	left ventricular
LVAD	left ventricular assist device
LVEF	left ventricular ejection fraction
MET	metabolic equivalent
MGE	multidmensional geriatric evaluation
MI	myocardial infarction
MICE	moderate-intensity continuous exercise
MVV	maximum voluntary ventilation
MWT	minute walk test
NYHA	New York Heart Association
PA	physical activity
PAD	peripheral artery disease
PCI	percutaneous coronary intervention
PDSA	Plan–Do–Study–Act
$PETCO_2$	end-tidal CO2 partial pressure
$PETO_2$	end-tidal O2 partial pressure
PHQ	Patient Health Questionnaire

PI	inspiratory mouth pressure
PM	pacemaker
PPG	photoplethysmography
RAMIT	Rehabilitation After Myocardial Infarction Trial
RCP	respiratory compensation point
RCT	randomized controlled trial
RD	risk difference
ReDS	remote dielectric sensing
RER	respiratory exchange ratio
RF	risk factor
RM	repetition management
RPE	rate of perceived exertion
RR	risk ratio
RT	resistance training
RTW	return to work
SDM	shared decision-making
SNRI	serotonin norepinephrine reuptake inhibitor
SOP	standard operating procedure
SPE	Scale of Perceived Exertion
SPPB	Short Physical Performance Battery
SSRI	selective serotonin reuptake inhibitor
STEMI	ST elevation myocardial infarction
TAVI	transcatheter aortic valve implantation
teleCR	tele-rehabilitation
UA	uric acid
VAD	ventricular assist device
VE	maximal ventilation
VO_2	oxygen consumption
VO_2/HR	oxygen pulse
VT	ventilatory threshold

Chapter 1

Evidence for cardiac rehabilitation in the modern era

Constantinos H. Davos and Bernhard Rauch

Summary

Management of cardiovascular disease (CVD) has rapidly improved during recent decades, and is still changing with the introduction of novel medication and advanced invasive procedures and devices. Notwithstanding these developments, cardiac rehabilitation (CR) is still a cornerstone of secondary prevention. Its effectiveness in improving the physical condition of chronic coronary syndrome (CCS) patients is beyond doubt, but its effectiveness on extending life expectancy is still a matter of debate. This chapter provides insights into the latest evidence (mainly presented in a recent meta-analysis of randomized controlled trials (RCTs) or controlled cohort studies) on the role of CR on morbidity and mortality in patients after an acute coronary event.

Introduction

CR is considered a fundamental strategy in the prevention of secondary CVD. It has received a class IA recommendation in European and international guidelines for improving outcome in patients after an acute coronary event or revascularization procedure. As many of the RCTs supporting this recommendation have been of small size with limited follow-up periods, the effect of CR on morbidity and mortality has mainly been evaluated by meta-analyses.

The evidence

The first meta-analyses by Oldridge et al. [1] and O'Connor et al. [2] were published more than 30 years ago, and included 10–22 RCTs with more than 4300 participants. These meta-analyses showed that exercise-based CR may lead to a 20–25% reduction in all-cause and CVD mortality compared with standard care methods. Subsequently, the effect of CR on clinical outcome was evaluated in a series of Cochrane systematic reviews. Cochrane publications are established as a highly reliable tool for assessment of scientific evidence with respect to the effectiveness of clinical interventions because of the extended systematic literature searches under-taken, the rigorous study selection and evaluation, and their improved statistical methodology. Therefore Cochrane meta-analyses often serve as the basis for clinical recommendations and guidelines.

The first Cochrane meta-analysis on the clinical effect of CR by Jolliffe et al. [3] was published in 2001, and subsequently updated by Taylor et al. (2004) [4] and Heran et al. (2011) [5]. The results of these Cochrane meta-analyses did not significantly change during this 10-year period, and showed that exercise-based CR may reduce all-cause mortality by 13–27% and CV mortality by 26–36%. However, despite their professionalism, accuracy, and completeness, these meta-analyses have been criti-cized for including RCTs of doubtful size and quality, in which women, the elderly, and high-risk populations were poorly represented. It has also been argued that the introduction of statins, angiotensin-converting enzyme (ACE) inhibitors, and dual anti-platelet therapy, as well as modern invasive techniques and devices, has changed the clinical course of coronary artery disease (CAD) in recent years, leading to significantly lower mortality after acute CAD events [6]. However, lower baseline mortality may significantly influence the efficacy of traditional therapeutic tools as represented by CR after acute coronary syndromes (ACS). Therefore, extrapolation of data on CR effectiveness obtained before the implementation of modern thera-peutic options may lead to considerable bias. As a consequence, the impression has arisen that the actual benefit of exercise-based CR may be largely overestimated.

Addressing these doubts, the most recent Cochrane review was published in 2016 by Anderson et al. [7] (Table 1.1). A significant reduction in CV mortality (10.4–7.6%) and hospitalization (30.7–26.1%) compared with controls was dem-onstrated in the exercise-based CR group. However, total mortality or the risk of fatal or non-fatal myocardial infarction (MI), coronary artery bypass grafting (CABG) procedures, or percutaneous coronary intervention (PCI) did not differ between the study groups. With respect to the case mix of the study populations, CR was particularly effective in reducing the CV mortality of post-MI patients but re-hospitalizations and PCI rates were unchanged. This Cochrane review also dis-tinguished between the subgroups of RCTs published before and after 1995, which showed an interesting result: CV mortality was significantly reduced by CR in both subgroups. However, a significant reduction in total mortality could only be shown in studies published before 1995.

The Rehabilitation After Myocardial Infarction Trial (RAMIT) attempted to address the lack of large prospective RCTs in this field, but failed to show a significant differ-ence in all-cause mortality between MI patients who were and were not referred to CR during 2 years of follow-up [8]. CR delivered in this study was comprehensive, including exercise training (ET) as the baseline intervention supplemented by health education and advice regarding secondary prevention. Unfortunately, RAMIT also had some serious limitations. The sample size was not large enough to reach a suf-ficient statistical power. Only 23% of the number of patients originally anticipated were enrolled in each group, and more than 20% of patients dropped out of the CR programme. Apart from this, the neutral result could be explained by the hetero-geneity of programmes and participating centres, resulting in variable doses of CR. The physical exercise dose during CR, the exercise intensity, and the number of CR sessions including exercise, information, education, and psychosocial support have

	Anderson et al, 2016 [7]	Rauch et al. 2016 [14]	van Halewijn et al. 2017 [12]	Sumner et al. 2017 [15]	Santiago de Araújo Pio et al. 2017 [11]	Abell et al. 2017 [17]	Powell et al. 2018 [18]
No. of trials	63	25	18	8	33	69	22
Literature search	Until July, 2014	1995 onwards	2010–15	2000 onwards	Until Nov. 2015	Until Jan. 2016	2000 onwards
No of participants	14 486	219 702	7691	9836	15 133	13 423	4834
Age	56 (median)	53.8–73.8	50–76	49.9–70.0	51.0–75.4	49–80	59.5 (mean)
Gender	<15% F	57–90% M	16–30% F	71–90% M	80.3% M	83% M	78.4% M
Population	MI, CABG or PCI, angina, CHD angiography defined	ACS (STEMI, NSTEMI, UA), CABG, mixed	MI, CABG or PCI, angina, CHD angiography defined	AMI (medically managed or revascularized)	Post-MI, HF, various cardiac diagnoses	CHD (ACS, HF, PCI, CABG, MI)	MI, CABG, PCI, angina, CHD defined by angiography
Study design	RCT	RCT, rCCS, pCCS	RCT	rCCS, pCCS	RCT, nRS, pOS, rOS (reporting CR dose)	RCT	RCT
Minimum follow-up	6 months	6 months	6 months	3 months	6 months	3 months	6 months
Follow-up	12 months (median)	40 months (mean)	24 months (median)	3–24 months	2 years (mean)	3 years (median)	24 weeks – 10 years 24.7months (mean)

Table 1.1 Most recent meta-analyses on the effects of cardiac rehabilitation

(continued)

Table 1.1 Continued

	Anderson et al. 2016 [7]	Rauch et al. 2016 [14]	van Halewijn et al. 2017 [12]	Sumner et al. 2017 [15]	Santiago de Araújo Pio et al. 2017 [11]	Abell et al. 2017 [17]	Powell et al. 2018 [18]
Intervention	EBCR (supervised/ unsupervised ExTr alone or with psychosocial and/ or educational interventions)	Supervised multi-component CR Start <3 months after discharge ExTr ≥2 times/ week plus at least one of: information, motivational techniques, education, psychological support & interventions, social and vocational support	CV prevention and CR (ExTr and/ or lifestyle based programme with at least one face-to-face session between healthcare provider and patient)	Supervised/ unsupervised, structured multi-component CR with ExTr and/or structured physical activity plus at least one of information provision, education, health behaviour change, psycho-logical support or intervention, social support.	Comprehensive CR CR dose subgroups Low: 4-11 sessions Medium: 12–35 sessions High: ≥36 sessions	EBCR with structured ExTr (supervised or unsupervised), with or without lifestyle modification and counseling	Supervised or unsupervised ExTr alone or as part of a comprehensive CR programme (educational/ psychosocial components)
Setting	Inpatient/ outpatient/ community-based/ home-based	Centre-based CR: inpatient/ outpatient/ mixed/teleCR		Inpatient/outpatient/ community-based/ home-based	Outpatient (≥4 sessions of structured ExTr plus at least patient education) Supervised (hospital-based/ medical-centre-based) and/or unsupervised (home-based/ community-based)	Any (home-based/ community-based/ outpatient centre based)	Hospital-based/ community-/ home-based

Control	Standard medical care and psychosocial and/or educational interventions, not structured ExTr	No CR participation	Usual care	No CR participation	Usual care (no CR dose)	Usual care	Standard medical care (optimal medical therapy, education, advice on diet and exercise, psychosocial support, no formal ExTr)
Results							
Total mortality	No effect	Reduced:* ACS: (pCCS: HR 0.37; rCCS: HR 0.64) CABG:(rCCS: HR 0.62) Mixed:(rCCS: HR 0.52)	Reduced only in comprehensive CR programmes managing ≥6 risk factors (RR 0.63)	Reduced (unadjusted OR 0.25; adjusted OR 0.47)	Low dose: No effect Medium dose: reduced (RR 0.58) High dose: reduced (RR 0.56)	Reduced RR 0.90, up to 10 years No effect up to 19 years	No effect
CV mortality	Reduced (RR 0.74)		Reduced (RR 0.42)	Reduced (unadjusted OR 0.21; adjusted OR: 0.43)	No effect	Reduced (RR 0.74 up to 10y, RR 0.87 up to 19y)	No effect
Recurrent MI	No effect (fatal and/or non-fatal)		Reduced (RR 0.70)	Reduced (unadjusted OR: 0.31)	No effect (non-fatal MI)	Reduced (RR 0.80 up to 10 years)	No effect

(continued)

Table 1.1 Continued

	Anderson et al, 2016 [7]	Rauch et al. 2016 [14]	van Halewijn et al. 2017 [12]	Sumner et al. 2017 [15]	Santiago de Araújo Pio et al. 2017 [11]	Abell et al. 2017 [17]	Powell et al. 2018 [18]
Hospital admissions	Reduced (RR 0.82)	No effect		No effect	No effect		Borderline reduction
Cerebro-vascular events			Reduced (RR 0.40)				
CABG	No effect				No effect Reduced in high dose (RR 0.60)	No effect	
Revasculari-zation	No effect			No effect	Reduced in high dose (RR 0.65)	No effect	

*For clarity 95% confidence intervals are not given.

If not otherwise noted all results arepresented as HR, OR, RR represent statistically significance.

ACS, acute coronary syndrome; (A)MI, (acute) myocardial infarction; CABG: coronary artery bypass grafting; CHD, coronary heart disease; CV, cardiovascular; EBCR, exercise-based cardiac rehabilitation; ExTr, exercise training; F, female; HF, heart failure; HR, hazards ratio; M, male; nRS, non-randomized studies; (n)STEMI, (non)ST elevation myocardial infarction; pCCS, prospective control cohort studies; PCI, percutaneous coronary interventions; pOS, prospective observational studies; rCCS, randomized control cohort studies; RCT, randomized control trials; rOS, randomized observational studies; RR, relative risk; UA, unstable angina.

been shown to be essential for CR success. Thus, RAMIT missed the opportunity of providing an undisputed answer to the effects of CR on patient mortality.

Importantly, the effectiveness of CR provided in everyday clinical practice is determined by the content, duration, intensity, and volume of exercise. This is in line with the observation that the physical fitness of patients in CR strongly correlates with mortality [9,10]. Accordingly, the Cochrane analysis convincingly showed that CR is particularly effective in reducing CV mortality or the re-infarction rate if the exercise volume delivered during CR exceeds a minimum [7]. Moreover, exercise intensity during CR should achieve the upper third of maximum oxygen consumption (VO_{2max}) or an equivalent measure [9,11], and all individual CV risks should consequently be addressed and treated [10,12].

Therefore, a minimum level of supervised and individually adjusted exercise volume is a basic requirement for CR to be successful in terms of improvement of clinical outcome. However, the content and features of CR often vary between and within different countries [13], and there are no internationally accepted minimum standards for evaluating the quality of CR delivery. The Cardiac Rehabilitation Outcomes Study (CROS) has been designed to take these inadequacies into account [14].

CROS was the first meta-analysis to include not only RCTs but also prospective and retrospective controlled cohort studies enrolling patients after ACS or CABG, or mixed populations with CAD. Studies were included in the subsequent meta-analysis only if the patients were participating in supervised comprehensive multidisciplinary CR starting no longer than three months after the index event and consisting of at least two weekly sessions of structured and supervised physical exercise. This should be supplemented by at least one of the following components: information, motivational techniques, education, psychological support and intervention, and social and vocational support. CROS investigated the effectiveness of CR on total mortality in the modern era of cardiology by only including studies published in 1995 or later, thereby reflecting the introduction of statin treatment and routine acute revascularization for treating ACS.

Apart from the RAMIT trial, no other RCT satisfied the CROS inclusion criteria, indicating that RCTs included in previous meta-analyses were mainly 'exercise-only CR studies' or were performed in the era before modern CAD treatment. CROS was the first meta-analysis to show a significant reduction in total mortality for CR participants after an ACS or CABG and in mixed CAD populations beyond the beneficial effects of modern medication (i.e. statins) and therapeutic procedures (i.e. acute coronary revascularization). For the first time, mortality reduction was also related to some minimal standards of CR delivery, which must be structured and multicomponent, including not only physical exercise but also educational sessions and psychosocial interventions, and must start early after the acute event (Table 1.1).

In line with the results of CROS were the results of the meta-analysis by Sumner et al. [15] which included eight observational studies published after the year 2000, enrolling acute MI patients. All-cause and cardiac mortality were reduced in the CR arm. As in CROS, no effect on re-hospitalization was found. The results of a later study by van Halewijn et al. [12], which included 18 RCTs with CAD patients published between 2010 and 2015, were able to elucidate these differences in morbidity and mortality. Based on the total study population, CV mortality, MIs and cerebrovascular events were reduced, but all-cause mortality was not. However, a significant reduction of all-cause mortality was observed under the condition that comprehensive CR programmes managed six or more CV risk factors (RFs) during the intervention, thus demonstrating the augmented effectiveness of the comprehensive CR by consequently addressing and treating all individual CV RFs. This finding was in line with the results of a previous meta-analysis by Lawler et al. [16] who showed that, in post-MI patients, only comprehensive CR could reduce total and cardiac mortality compared with exercise-based CR alone. In this study, CR was only associated with a significant reduction of cardiac mortality if its duration exceeded three months, again highlighting the role of CR dose. Further, a recent meta-analysis by Santiago de Araújo Pio et al. [11] demonstrated that total mortality reduction was only feasible in CVD patients who participated in medium- and high-dose CR sessions (Table 1.1) [11]. Another CR component, the level of adherence to the exercise intervention, was the only covariate affecting total mortality (28% relative risk reduction) and CV mortality (28% relative risk reduction) in a meta-regression analysis by Abell et al. [17] which included RCTs performed until 2017 enrolling participants with diverse CAD diagnoses (Table 1.1). Total mortality was significantly reduced in the exercised-based CR group within a follow-up period of 10 years, but this effect was not sustained during an extended follow-up period of 19 years. However, the significant reduction in CV mortality observed in this study was maintained over the whole follow-up period of 19 years.

The most recent meta-analysis by Powell et al. [18] focused on a re-evaluation of the Cochrane analysis by restricting the study inclusion period to the year 2000 onwards and including RCTs with zero events during follow-up (Table 1.1). Risk ratios (RRs) or risk differences (RDs) were calculated. No significant differences between the study groups could be detected under these conditions. However, the serious methodological limitations of this meta-analysis hamper a sound interpretation of the results. Thirteen studies (out of 22) investigated a mixed population, including stable CAD patients, and differentiation of patients with acute CV events initiating CR delivery (e.g. ACS or CABG) was not possible. Only one of the six studies including ACS patients satisfied the minimal inclusion criteria of CROS [14]. The preconditions for a successful CR, as discussed previously, were not sufficiently taken into account, and internationally accepted requirements for the biometric evaluation of zero-event studies were not followed [19,20]. Finally, the most recent update of CROS (CROS II) reconfirmed the effectiveness of CR participation after ACS or CABG in actual clinical practice by reducing total mortality in patients under evidence-based medical treatment [21].

Conclusion

The most important reason for practising evidence-based medicine is to improve the quality of healthcare by identifying clinically effective practices, while rejecting those that are ineffective. Although meta-analyses are not infallible and may include studies with high heterogeneity in design, quality, and quantity of CR delivered, they contain important information on CR effectiveness. They provide evidence that exercise-based CR may reduce CV mortality and all-cause mortality after ACS or CABG in the modern era of revascularization and medication. In particular, reduction of

Table 1.2 Minimal requirements for successful cardiac rehabilitation derived from recent meta-analyses

Intervention	Supervised multicomponent cardiac rehabilitation
Start	Within 3 months after discharge
Setting	Any (inpatient/outpatient/community-based/home-based/mixed/tele-rehabilitation)
Exercise components	<ul><li>*Frequency:* ≥ 2 times/week</li><li>*Duration:* > 3 months</li><li>≥ 36 sessions</li><li>*Intensity:* upper third of VO_{2max}</li><li>≥1000 units (no. of exercise weeks × average no. of sessions/week × average duration of session in minutes)</li></ul>
Other components	<ul><li>At least once a week: information, motivational techniques, education, psychological support and interventions, social and vocational support</li><li>Management of six or more of the following risk factors: smoking cessation, physical exercise training, counselling for exercise/activity, diet, blood pressure, cholesterol, glucose levels, checking medication, stress management</li></ul>

mortality could be achieved if CR starts early after the acute coronary event and is structured, multicomponent, and delivered by an organized team of qualified health professionals. The duration of CR, the exercise dose, and the adherence to CR are important parameters in achieving these favourable effects (Table 1.2). However, further evidence is needed regarding endpoints such as re-hospitalization, non-fatal MI, and revascularization.

References

1. Oldridge NB, Guyatt GH, Fischer ME, Rimm AA. Cardiac rehabilitation after myocardial infarction. Combined experience of randomized clinical trials. *JAMA* 1988; 260: 945–50.
2. O'Connor GT, Buring JE, Yusuf S, et al. An overview of randomized trials of rehabilitation with exercise after myocardial infarction. *Circulation* 1989; 80: 234–44.
3. Jolliffe JA, Rees K, Taylor RS, et al. Exercise-based rehabilitation for coronary heart disease. *Cochrane Database Syst Rev* 2000; (4): CD001800.
4. Taylor RS, Brown A, Ebrahim S, et al. Exercise-based rehabilitation for patients with coronary heart disease: systematic review and meta-analysis of randomized controlled trials. *Am J Med* 2004; 116: 682–92.
5. Heran BS, Chen JM, Ebrahim S, et al. Exercise-based cardiac rehabilitation for coronary heart disease. *Cochrane Database Syst Rev* 2011; (7): CD001800.
6. Puymirat E, Simon T, Cayla G, et al. Acute myocardial infarction: changes in patient characteristics, management, and 6-month outcomes over a period of 20 years in the FAST-MI program (French

Registry of Acute ST-Elevation or Non-ST-Elevation Myocardial Infarction) 1995 to 2015. *Circulation* 2017; 136: 1908–19.

7. Anderson L, Thompson DR, Oldridge N, et al. Exercise-based cardiac rehabilitation for coronary heart disease. *Cochrane Database Syst Rev* 2016;(1): CD001800.

8. West RR, Jones DA, Henderson AH. Rehabilitation After Myocardial Infarction Trial (RAMIT): multicentre randomized controlled trial of comprehensive cardiac rehabilitation in patients following myocardial infarction. *Heart* 2012; 98: 637–44.

9. Kavanagh T, Mertens DJ, Hamm LF, et al. Peak oxygen intake and cardiac mortality in women referred for cardiac rehabilitation. *J Am Coll Cardiol* 2003; 42: 2139–43.

10. Martin BJ, Arena R, Haykowsky M, et al. Cardiovascular fitness and mortality after contemporary cardiac rehabilitation. *Mayo Clin Proc* 2013; 88: 455–63.

11. Santiago de Araújo Pio C, Marzolini S, Pakosh M, Grace SL. Effect of cardiac rehabilitation dose on mortality and morbidity: a systematic review and meta-regression analysis. *Mayo Clin Proc* 2017; 92: 1644–59.

12. van Halewijn G, Deckers J, Tay HY, et al. Lessons from contemporary trials of cardiovascular prevention and rehabilitation: a systematic review and meta-analysis. *Int J Cardiol* 2017; 232: 294–303.

13. Benzer W, Rauch B, Schmid JP, et al. Exercise-based cardiac rehabilitation in twelve European countries results of the European Cardiac Rehabilitation Registry. *Int J Cardiol* 2017; 228: 58–67.

14. Rauch B, Davos CH, Doherty P, et al. The prognostic effect of cardiac rehabilitation in the era of acute revascularisation and statin therapy: a systematic review and meta-analysis of randomized and non-randomized studies—the Cardiac Rehabilitation Outcome Study (CROS). *Eur J Prev Cardiol* 2016; 23: 1914–39.

15. Sumner J, Harrison A, Doherty P. The effectiveness of modern cardiac rehabilitation: a systematic review of recent observational studies in non-attenders versus attenders. *PLoS One* 2017; 12: e0177658.

16. Lawler PR, Filion KB, Eisenberg MJ. Efficacy of exercise-based cardiac rehabilitation post-myocardial infarction: a systematic review and meta-analysis of randomized controlled trials. *Am Heart J* 2011; 162: 571–84.e2.

17. Abell B, Glasziou P, Hoffmann T. The contribution of individual exercise training components to clinical outcomes in randomised controlled trials of cardiac rehabilitation: a systematic review and meta-regression. *Sports Med Open* 2017; 3: 19.

18. Powell R, McGregor G, Ennis S, et al. Is exercise-based cardiac rehabilitation effective? A systematic review and meta-analysis to re-examine the evidence. *BMJ Open* 2018; 8(3): e019656.

19. Bradburn MJ, Deeks JJ, Berlin JA, Russell Localio A. Much ado about nothing: a comparison of the performance of meta-analytical methods with rare events. *Stat Med* 2007; 26: 53–77.

20. Lane PW. Meta-analysis of incidence of rare events. *Stat Methods Med Res* 2013; 22: 117–32.

21. Salzwedel A, Jensen K, Rauch B, et al. Effectiveness of comprehensive cardiac rehabilitation in coronary artery disease patients treated according to contemporary evidence based medicine. Update of the Cardiac Rehabilitation Outcome Study (CROS-II). *Eur J Prev Cardiol* 2020; 23 February:2047487320905719.

Further reading

Ambrosetti M, Abreu A, Corrà U, et al. Secondary prevention through comprehensive cardiac rehabilitation: from knowledge to implementation. 2020 update. A position paper from the Secondary Prevention and Rehabilitation Section of the European Association of Preventive Cardiology. *Eur J Prev Cardiol* 2020; 30 March: 2047487320913379.

Piepoli MF, Corrà U, Abreu A, et al. Challenges in secondary prevention of cardiovascular diseases: a review of the current practice. *Int J Cardiol* 2015; 180: 114–19.

Piepoli MF, Hoes AW, Agewall S, et al. European Guidelines on cardiovascular disease prevention in clinical practice: The Sixth Joint Task Force of the European Society of Cardiology and Other Societies on Cardiovascular Disease Prevention in Clinical Practice. *Eur Heart J* 2016; 37: 2315–81.

Chapter 2

Different settings for cardiac rehabilitation

Jean-Paul Schmid and Ugo Corrà

Summary

Cardiac rehabilitation (CR) has traditionally been viewed as a hospital-based intervention consisting of a multidisciplinary exercise-based programme, aimed at improving exercise capacity after an acute CV event or surgery and optimizing the CV risk profile. Because of various limitations on attendance at these programmes, in particular lack of availability or difficulties in accessibility, alternative settings for providing secondary preventive measures have been developed. Amongst them, home-based rehabilitation with or without telemonitoring has the potential to increase patient participation and support behavioural changes. This may be a reasonable option for selected clinically stable patients at low to moderate risk who are eligible for CR but cannot attend a traditional hospital- or centre-based CR programme. Although short-term improvements in functional capacity, health-related quality of life (HRQoL), and CV risk factor control are comparable in home-based and hospital- or centre-based CR, long-term studies of the impact of home-based CR on clinical events are still needed.

Introduction

Increasing awareness of the negative impact of mobility restriction (six weeks of bed rest in the 1930s) and chair therapy (in the 1940s) as well as concerns about the safety of unsupervised exercise in patients with acute coronary events led to the development of simple monitored exercise programmes. Initially, safe resumption of physical activity (PA) and return to work (RTW) were the primary aims of CR, but in the 1950s Hellerstein introduced the concept of comprehensive CR, which was eventually adopted in CR programmes worldwide [1].

Since then, CR has evolved further towards multidisciplinary programmes, mostly based in hospitals or health centres, focusing on risk factor (RF) management, optimization of medical treatment, nutritional counselling, smoking cessation, and psychosocial care. They are based on the definition of rehabilitation by the World Health Organization (WHO), namely offering a 'sum of activities that should aim to influence favourably the underlying cause of the disease, as well as to ensure the patient the best possible physical, mental and social conditions, so that they may, by their own efforts, preserve or resume, when lost, as normal a place as possible in the life of the community'. In recent times, home-based CR programmes have been proposed as an alternative to classical hospital- or centre-based programmes, thus overcoming some of the barriers to traditional CR participation.

Organization of cardiac rehabilitation

Traditionally, CR is divided into three phases [2]. Phase I, or the inpatient phase, applies to the post-acute phase when the patient is still in hospital. It consists of early progressive mobilization of the stable cardiac patient to the level of activity required to leave hospital and perform simple tasks of daily living. The progressive reduction of the duration of hospital stay in modern cardiology precludes conducting a formal inpatient education and training programme. Thus phase I rehabilitation is mostly limited to early mobilization (EM), brief counselling about the nature of the illness, treatment, RF management, and follow-up planning, in which it is imperative to include referral to phase II CR.

Phase II corresponds to a structured, multidisciplinary, supervised programme aiming at further improvement of physical performance and, even more importantly, implementing all necessary secondary preventive measures to improve long-term prognosis. Secondary prevention through exercise-based CR is the intervention with the best scientific evidence for contributing to decreases in morbidity and mortality following cardiac interventions or chronic disease states such as chronic coronary syndromes or stable heart failure (HF). Practical recommendations for the core components and aims of CR intervention in various CV conditions are well summarized by Piepoli et al. [3]. Phase II CR is usually offered as hospital- or centre-based ambulatory outpatient CR programme with a duration of 2–6 months. Residential programmes of 3–4 weeks duration are also available in some countries.

Phase III is a lifetime maintenance phase in which physical fitness and additional RF reduction are emphasized. It consists of home- or gymnasium-based exercise, mostly led by qualified personnel.

Alternative models of cardiac rehabilitation

Despite its proven benefits, CR referral and participation rates remain low. Reasons are manifold and differences in healthcare policies and delivery systems between countries may play a role. However, barriers raised by healthcare providers and patients themselves also exist (Table 2.1) [4].

These challenges have led to the development of a large number of alternative models of CR [5]. The most important of these are as follows:
a) Multifactorial individualized telehealth delivery addresses many RFs and provides individualized assessment and RF modification, mostly by telephone contact.

Table 2.1 Patient, healthcare provider, and health system based barriers to implementation of secondary prevention measures

Patient	Clinician/healthcare provider	Healthcare system
Medication side-effects	Failure to initiate treatment	Lack of clinical guidelines
Too many medications	Failure to titrate to goal	Lack of care coordination
Cost of medications	Failure to set clear goals	No visit planning
Denial of disease	Underestimation of patient need	Lack of decision support
Denial of disease severity	Failure to identify and manage comorbid conditions	Poor communication between physician and others involved in the patient's healthcare provision
Forgetfulness	Insufficient time	No disease registry
Perception of low susceptibility	Insufficient focus of emphasis on goal attainment	No active outreach
Absence of disease symptoms	Reactive rather than proactive	Perverse incentives
Poor communication with physician	Poor communication skills	Pressure to shorten length of hospital stay
Mistrust of physician	Shortage of time	Healthcare systems focused on acute care (hospital-based health systems)
Depression, mental disease, substance abuse	Poor awareness of value of preventive measure	Lack of preventive structure
Poor health literacy/poor awareness of value of preventive measure		Poorly designed preventive programmes/lack of quality control

Reproduced from Piepoli MF, Corra U, Dendale P, et al. Challenges in secondary prevention after acute myocardial infarction: A call for action. *Eur J Prev Cardiol* 2016;23:1994-2006. with permission from SAGE Publishing.

b) Internet-based delivery: most patient–provider contact for RF modification is via the internet.
c) Telehealth interventions focusing on exercise: mostly by telephone contact, often including the use of telemonitoring.
d) Telehealth interventions focusing on recovery: mostly by telephone contact. The intervention content is focused on supporting psychosocial recovery from an acute cardiac event such as MI or CABG.

e) Community- or home-based CR: mostly delivered face-to-face via either home visits or patient attendance at community centres (for programmes other than traditional CR).

f) Programmes specific to rural, remote, and culturally and linguistically diverse populations.

g) Multiple models of care: multifaceted interventions across a number of these categories.

h) Complementary and alternative medicine interventions.

However, clinical studies have shown that only the community- and telehealth-based individualized and multifactorial models for CR are associated with improvements in CVD RF profile comparable with those obtained using the traditional hospital- or centre-based approach. Therefore, in the most recent European Guidelines on CV disease prevention in clinical practice, alternative rehabilitation models are rated as follows [6].

a) Home-based rehabilitation with or without telemonitoring holds promise for increasing participation and supporting behavioural change.

b) Home-based rehabilitation programmes have the potential to increase patient participation by offering greater flexibility and options for activities.

Home-based CR can be carried out in a variety of settings, including the home or other non-clinical settings such as community centres, health clubs, and parks. The main advantage is to overcome geographic, logistical, and other access-related barriers. Furthermore, home-based CR has the potential to expand the breadth and depth of educational, counselling, and monitoring options for patients because of its unrestricted availability in time, compared with the 3–4 hours weekly of personal contact with staff in hospital-based rehabilitation. Potential advantages and disadvantages of home-based CR are listed in Table 2.2.

Table 2.2 Potential advantages and disadvantages of home-based CR	
Advantages	Disadvantages
Reduced enrolment delays	Lack of reimbursement
Expanded capacity/access	Less intensive ET
Individually tailored programmes	Less social support
Flexible and convenient scheduling	Less patient accountability
Minimal travel/transportation barriers	Lack of published standards
Greater privacy while receiving CR services	Less face-to-face monitoring and communication
Integration with regular home routine	Safety concerns for patients at higher risk

Reproduced from Thomas RJ, Beatty AL, Beckie TM, et al. Home-Based Cardiac Rehabilitation: A Scientific Statement From the American Association of Cardiovascular and Pulmonary Rehabilitation, the American Heart Association, and the American College of Cardiology. *Journal of the American College of Cardiology* 2019;74(1):133–153. DOI: 10.1016/j.jacc.2019.03.008 with permission from Elsevier.

The core components of home-based cardiac rehabilitation

Hospital-based, centre-based, and home-based CR all adopt a systematic, multidisciplinary, and team-based approach to patient-centred care, including behavioural counselling and patient activation which are promoted through multiple individualized interactions with patients over time. These include management of lipids, blood pressure (BP), diabetes mellitus (DM), and cardioprotective medication. It is important that the core components of hospital- and centre-based CR, i.e. patient assessment, exercise training, dietary counselling, RF management, and psychosocial interventions, are also included in home-based CR services.

Whereas most hospital- or centre-based CR programmes are supervised, group-based, and partially monitored by telemetry, home-based CR involves walking with variable support via telephone calls or home visits from a physical therapist, exercise physiologist, or nurse. Provision of home exercise equipment may be considered for some patients who are unable to walk briskly or jog because of comorbid conditions or logistical barriers (e.g. lack of access to a safe walking surface or gym). The provision of home exercise treadmills or stationary cycles plus a heart rate (HR) monitor may be associated with increased adherence to regular exercise.

In the home-based setting, dietary information can be conveyed via telephone, weekly educational and counselling meetings (including practice cooking sessions), home visits, educational materials, or a web portal or smartphone.

Psychosocial support principles of goal setting and motivational interviewing should also be applied, as well as education on medication. Smoking cessation strategies are a particularly important component of CR services, and the use of home-based and mobile health delivery models of smoking cessation should be considered.

Regarding the need for adjustments in preventive medications, close coordination of care between the CR staff and the patient's physician is critically important.

Effects of home-based cardiac rehabilitation compared with hospital- or centre-based cardiac rehabilitation

Lifestyle changes that occur during hospital- or centre-based CR may deteriorate when these interventions are withdrawn [7]. It is possible that the higher degree of self-monitoring, management, and unsupervised exercise inherent in home-based CR programmes may make the transition from active intervention to lifelong disease self-management easier.

Severe CV events are rare in low- or moderate-risk patients. Nevertheless, a careful risk assessment should be carried out before starting home-based training, especially in higher-risk patients. Particular caution is warranted in the presence of typical clinical concerns of hypoglycaemia in diabetics, haemodynamic changes in patients with HF, and falls in older patients, or if higher-intensity training is aimed. Additional safety data are needed for home-based CR, particularly in higher-risk groups.

Adherence to CR therapy appears to be better in home-based CR than in hospital- or centre-based CR because of the greater flexibility and convenience for patients who use home-based CR services. However, a lack of reimbursement by most third-party payers is a challenge to home-based CR implementation.

Evidence-based standards and guidelines for hospital- and centre-based CR have been widely disseminated and can be readily adapted to home-based CR. Quality metrics for home-based CR, when developed, should focus on key structure, process, and outcome metrics.

Technological tools are advancing at a rapid pace and will help to improve communication between patients and providers, enhance the validity of patient monitoring for safety and effectiveness, and expand the reach of CR professionals beyond the typical hospital CR services towards the home-based setting.

Further research is recommended to assess the impact of home-based CR services in more diverse and higher-risk patient groups and the impact of hybrid models of CR, including specific components from hospital- or centre-based CR and home-based CR. Such information will support negotiations of reimbursement policies from third-party insurance providers, a critically important step in the implementation of home-based CR services.

Conclusion

Although the science behind home-based CR is relatively new and less developed than that for other CR settings, its findings are generally consistent with those reported for hospital- and centre-based CR. Available evidence suggests that home-based CR may provide an alternative option for CR services for stable CVD patients at low- to moderate-risk patients who cannot access hospital- or centre-based services. Technological tools are advancing at a rapid pace and may further facilitate the implementation of home-based CR. Shorter-term improvements in functional capacity, HRQol, and CVD risk factor control are similar in home-based and in hospital- or centre-based CR. However, longer-term studies of the impact of home-based CR on clinical events are still lacking.

References

1. Bethell HJ. Cardiac rehabilitation: from Hellerstein to the millennium. *Int J Clin Pract* 2000; 54: 92–7.

2. Mampuya WM. Cardiac rehabilitation past, present and future: an overview. *Cardiovasc Diagn Ther* 2012; 2: 38–49.

3. Piepoli MF, Corrà U, Benzer W, et al. Secondary prevention through cardiac rehabilitation: from knowledge to implementation. A position paper from the Cardiac Rehabilitation Section of the European Association of Cardiovascular Prevention and Rehabilitation. *Eur J Cardiovasc Prev Rehabil* 2010; 17: 1–17.

4. Piepoli MF, Corrà U, Dendale P, et al. Challenges in secondary prevention after acute myocardial infarction: a call for action. *Eur J Prev Cardiol* 2016; 23: 1994–2006.

5. Clark RA, Conway A, Poulsen V, et al. Alternative models of cardiac rehabilitation: a systematic review. *Eur J Prev Cardiol* 2015; 22: 35–74.

6. Piepoli MF, Hoes AW, Agewall S, et al. European Guidelines on cardiovascular disease prevention in clinical practice: the Sixth Joint Task Force of the European Society of Cardiology and Other Societies on Cardiovascular Disease Prevention in Clinical Practice. *Eur Heart J* 2016; 37: 2315–81.

7. Thomas RJ, Beatty AL, Beckie TM, et al. Home-based cardiac rehabilitation: a scientific statement from the American Association of Cardiovascular and Pulmonary Rehabilitation, the American Heart Association, and the American College of Cardiology. *J Am Coll Cardiol* 2019; 74: 133–53.

Further reading

Grace SL, Turk-Adawi KI, Contractor A, et al. Cardiac rehabilitation delivery model for low-resource settings. An International Council of Cardiovascular Prevention and Rehabilitation Consensus Statement. *Prog Cardiovasc Dis* 2016; 59: 303–22.

Nabutovsky I, Nachshon A, Klempfner R, et al. Digital cardiac rehabilitation programs: the future of patient-centered medicine. *Telemed J E Health*; 26: 34–41.

Chapter 3

Cardiac rehabilitation: referral and barriers

Massimo Francesco Piepoli and Margaret E. Cupples

Summary

For many patients with CVD, CR offers an important introduction to secondary prevention. However, many do not enjoy the benefits of CR, often because they are not referred. Internationally, levels of CR attendance vary; overall, less than half of those eligible to attend do so. Patients who are least likely to be referred may benefit most from attendance: structured referral systems increase referral rates. Barriers to CR uptake exist at the levels of patients (education; adherence to healthy lifestyle advice; adherence to medication), healthcare providers (knowledge and motivation; risk stratification; post-discharge plans; inter-professional communication), and healthcare systems (availability of structured programmes; referral processes; performance measures). Multilevel interdisciplinary interventions are required to address these barriers.

Introduction

Despite the availability of secondary prevention and CR programmes, many patients who might benefit from such programmes are not referred or fail to attend [1]. Across Europe, there is wide geographical variation in provision of CR [2] but several studies have shown how, whilst only about 50% of eligible patients are referred overall, approximately 80% of those who are referred do attend [3–5]. A recent observational study across 24 European countries (Euroaspire IV) [5] found that 51% of patients were advised to attend CR after a cardiac event; 81% of these attended at least half of the sessions, compared with 41% of the overall sample, and the proportion advised to attend varied from 0% to 85% across different countries.

Referral rates can be increased through electronic prompts or automatic systems, engaging nurses and therapists, and early post-discharge programmes. Increased referral, structured follow-up (liaison visit) and early outpatient education improve patient CR uptake [1,6,7]. One review concluded that the highest uptake was achieved by combining automatic referral with a liaison visit or motivational letter [8]. European guidelines on CVD prevention [9] provide evidence-based recommendations on referral to preventive programmes.

Women, ethnic minorities, older patients, and those with multiple comorbidities are less likely to participate in CR. A meta-analysis found that enrolment of women in CR was 36% less likely than for men [10]. However, combined systematic and liaison-facilitated referral resulted in significantly greater enrolment among women than non-systematic referral [11]. Although less likely to be referred, older patients may benefit more, and those with the lowest fitness at baseline may gain greatest benefit [12,13]. Patients in CR with low fitness (<5 metabolic equivalents (METs) on treadmill testing) had a 30% reduction in overall mortality at one year with each MET increase achieved at 12 weeks, compared with a 13% reduction for those with higher baseline fitness [12]. The patients with low fitness were older (28% aged >75 years) and had more comorbidities than those in other groups. Among older patients with HF (mean age, 78 years), 72% indicated that they would like to attend CR, although their preference for location and design varied, with 40% preferring a group-based programme (hospital-based, 25%; community-based, 15%), and 30% a home-based programme [14]. Approaches to maximize referral are important to optimize uptake of CR.

Barriers to CR uptake

A plethora of research indicates that patient, healthcare provider and/or health system based barriers share responsibility for suboptimal CR uptake and adherence [6] (Table 3.1).

Patient-related barriers

Patient-related barriers to CR include factors which affect their education and empowerment, adherence to healthy lifestyles, and adherence to preventive pharmacological therapy.

Many patients have a poor understanding of their disease and perceive themselves as having little control over its course; many lack interest in prevention and/or feel embarrassed about participating in CR group sessions [15]. Others report not receiving robust information and/or encouragement from health professionals regarding prevention of recurrent events [15,16]. Lack of social support, poor psychological wellbeing, inconvenient location, transport difficulties, competing work commitments, and financial cost also hinder CR attendance [16].

Inadequacies and time constraints regarding education and counselling lead to poor implementation of preventive care. Patients with a clear understanding of their after-hospital care are 30% less likely to be readmitted or to visit the emergency department after discharge than those who lack this information [17]. Patients discharged from hospital with a clear guideline-oriented treatment recommendation, a written checklist of measures to support risk modification and lifestyle change, education about self-care, and clear plans for follow-up can better understand the importance and potential impact of this information [18].

Adherence to healthy lifestyle advice is associated with reduced risk of recurrence of CV events [19] but is difficult for many patients. A recent study involving 131 centres in 27 countries found that, six months after a CVD event, 19% smoked, 38% were obese, and 34% failed to meet recommendations for physical activity (PA) [20].

Table 3.1	Patient, clinician, and healthcare system level barriers to CVD prevention and CR	
Patient	Clinician/healthcare provider	Healthcare system
Perception of low susceptibility	Underestimation of patient need	Lack of clinical guidelines
Absence of symptoms/denial of disease	Failure to initiate treatment	No disease registry Lack of decision support
Low health literacy/low awareness of value of preventive measures	Poor awareness of significance of risk/value of preventive measures	No active outreach Lack of preventive structure
Forgetfulness		No visit/review planning
Poor communication with physician	Poor communication skills/time limitations	Pressure of short hospital stay
Mistrust of physician	Failure to identify needs/priorities	Focus on acute care (hospital-based)
Low adherence to lifestyle advice	Failure to agree clear goals/monitor progress/provide support/review	Perverse incentives
Adverse social/environmental influences on healthy lifestyle	Inadequate proactive planning/poor recognition of external influences or patient's needs/poor inter-professional communication	Poor communication systems within/between health and social care structures
Comorbidities (e.g. depression, mental illness, substance abuse)	Poor management of comorbid conditions	Lack of care coordination
Low adherence to prescribed medication	Failure to communicate importance of medication for risk reduction	Poorly designed preventive programmes
Multiple medications, medication side effects, cost of medications	Failure to optimize medication and titrate to goal appropriately	Poor performance monitoring/quality control

A wide variety of techniques to support lifestyle change have been evaluated: self-monitoring of PA, action planning, and coping strategies appear helpful [21], alongside multisectoral initiatives [22].

A meta-analysis of adherence to cardio-protective medicines in >350 000 patients found low adherence in individuals at high CV risk (66%) and in patients with CVD (50%) a median of two years after initiating a prescription [23]. Lower adherence to medication has been shown to be associated with worse outcomes and higher healthcare costs [24]. Reasons for non-adherence are complex and include demographic, socio-economic and health systems factors, health literacy, intensity of follow-up and review, complex medication regimens, and adverse effects of therapy [25]. Healthcare providers should assess adherence, identify reasons for non-adherence, and provide personally tailored advice to promote adherence [9], whilst considering the development of real or presumed 'drug intolerance'.

A Cochrane review [26] of interventions to improve medication adherence advised involving allied professionals such as nurses and pharmacists in delivering interventions, which may include telephone follow-up, interim appointments, and monitoring of repeat prescriptions. Non-professionals within the patient's social context, including family members, carers, or lay groups in the community, may provide cost-effective support to improve adherence.

Cardiac patients may present with several comorbidities needing multiple treatments and sometimes interacting. The physician's role is to simplify treatment regimens to their lowest acceptable level, monitoring outcomes, and providing feedback [9]. Polypill or combination therapy may improve adherence to prescribed medication. 'Medicines optimization' may mean de-prescribing: evaluating when to discontinue medicines (e.g. stopping long-term beta-blocker post MI in patients without a specific indication) is important.

Healthcare provider barriers

Healthcare provider barriers relate to knowledge and motivation, risk stratification, post-discharge planning, and inter-professional communication.

The ESC defines the knowledge needed by cardiologists regarding secondary prevention and CR, including evaluation and management of CV risk [27]. However, such requirements may not be included in the curriculum of all cardiologists or specialist allied health professionals. This knowledge gap should be closed by specific educational training. Patients who participate in CR consistently cite physicians and other healthcare providers as their main sources of encouragement [16].

For decades, providers have been encouraged to shift care away from inpatient hospital stays toward less expensive outpatient treatment [28]. Among the metrics for gauging the success of this endeavour is early discharge and a shorter hospital stay, although its cost-effectiveness is uncertain and it limits the time available for providing education, risk stratification, and secondary prevention therapy before discharge. Risk stratification is a prerequisite for improving care management. Current guidelines recommend evaluation of metabolic risk markers during the index admission; as the risk of events decreases with time, early assessment (e.g. infarct size, resting left ventricular function) is crucial [9].

Strategies to improve CR uptake include provision of patient education, structured follow-up via telephone, healthcare professional visit, or both, gender-tailored sessions, a specific programme for older patients, and planned early appointments for programmes [1,7,9,29]. Timely transfer of specialist knowledge from hospital-based healthcare professionals to those based in the community remains a major challenge. Delayed or inaccurate communication between healthcare professionals has substantial implications for continuity of care, patient safety, patient and clinician satisfaction, and resource use. Educational meetings, audit, feedback with local opinion leaders, and computer decision support devices can lead to improved continuity of care [29].

Regular review and provision of patient education leads to improved adherence to lifestyle advice (more PA, better diet), reduced symptoms, improved HRQol, and reduced mortality [30]. In some countries, clinical indicators of general practitioner (GP) performance in chronic disease monitoring have included checklists relating to medication and RF control, with engagement in this process being incentivized by financial reward [31].

Healthcare systems barriers

Unfortunately, the lack of structured CR programmes, referral processes, and measures of performance may have a negative influence on referral rates within healthcare systems.

The lack of prevention centres is an obstacle to implementation of rehabilitation programmes in many European countries, particularly in less financially advantaged regions [32]. Inter-hospital variability in referral rates suggests the influence of healthcare system factors, including insurance coverage and hospital characteristics (size, geographic location). Limited financial incentives and competing workload priorities may have a negative influence on referral rates [33]. However, it is recognized that implementing systematic processes can increase referral rates by more than 50%, and the strength of physician endorsement is a pivotal step in improving participation, associated with improved outcomes after MI [16].

Table 3.2. Examples of patient, provider, and system level interventions to improve CR uptake

Intervention	Description of intervention
Patient level • Education: patient decision aids • Patient organizations • Self-management	Provide information (verbal, written, media, web): treatment options and outcomes Partnership working: patients, carers and clinicians sharing information Self-monitoring: medication decisions made with healthcare provider support
Provider level • Educational meetings • Audit and feedback • Educational outreach visits • Local opinion leaders • Computer-assisted decision support	Conferences, lectures, workshops, seminars, symposia: promote guidelines Summary (written, verbal, or electronic) of clinical performance over a time period 'Face-to-face' visits by trained person to health professionals (academic detailing) Healthcare professionals considered by colleagues as 'educationally influential' Automated clinical decision advice based on individual patient data
Organizational/system level • Clinical pathways • Financial incentives • Legislation	Automatic CR referral; structured multidisciplinary care plans for specific problems Based on service, episode, or visit; related to level of provision/quality of care Smoking bans; population-level restrictions

Source data from Nieuwlaat R. Schwalm JD, Khatib R, et al. Why are we failing to implement effective therapies in cardiovascular disease? *Eur Heart J* 2013;34:1262-69.

The lack of benefit from some interventions [34] highlights the need for quality and minimum standards in preventive programmes. Audit of programmes should include information about the core components and their implementation, clinical outcomes, and patient satisfaction. Accountability measures, including referral, performance/quality indicators (e.g. percentage of patients referred or prescription of evidence-based medications [31]), and financial incentives for performance should increase the willingness of physicians to refer and improve the delivery of prevention. Benchmarking against local, regional, and national standards provides measures of performance and quality for commissioners of services.

Conclusion

Improving CR participation requires action at a number of levels including legislation, international and national guidelines, and local strategies [2,6,29]. Interventions which support engagement in CR may target patients, providers, and healthcare systems (Table 3.2). These approaches should be tailored to implementation in specific situations, taking account of current performance measures.

References

1. Karmali KN, Davies P, Taylor F, et al. Promoting patient uptake and adherence in cardiac rehabilitation. *Cochrane Database Syst Rev* 2014; (6); CD007131.

2. Bjarnason-Wehrens B, McGee H, Zwisler A-D, et al. Cardiac rehabilitation in Europe: results from the European Cardiac Rehabilitation Inventory Survey. *Eur J Prev Cardiol* 2010; 17: 410–18.

3. Cupples ME, Tully MA, Dempster M, et al. Cardiac rehabilitation uptake following myocardial infarction: cross-sectional study in primary care. *Br J Gen Pract* 2010; 60: 431–5.

4. Kotseva K, Wood D, De Backer G, De Bacquer D. Use and effects of cardiac rehabilitation in patients with coronary heart disease: results from the EUROASPIRE III survey. *Eur J Prev Cardiol* 2012; 20: 817–26.

5. Kotseva K, Wood D, De Bacquer D, et al. Determinants of participation and risk factor control according to attendance in cardiac rehabilitation programmes in coronary patients in Europe: EUROASPIRE IV survey. *Eur J Prev Cardiol* 2018; 12: 1242–51.

6. Clark AM, King-Shier KM, Duncan A, et al. Factors influencing referral to cardiac rehabilitation and secondary prevention programs: a systematic review. *Eur J Prev Cardiol* 2012; 20: 692–700.

7. Grace SL, Angevaare KL, Reid RD, et al. Effectiveness of inpatient and outpatient strategies in increasing referral and utilisation of cardiac rehabilitation: a prospective, multi-site study. *Implement Sci* 2012; 7: 120–7.

8. Gravely-Witte S, Leung YW, Nariani R, et al. Effects of cardiac rehabilitation referral strategies on referral and enrollment rates. *Nat Rev Cardiol* 2010; 7: 87–96.

9. Piepoli MF, Hoes AW, Agewall S, et al. European Guidelines on cardiovascular disease prevention in clinical practice. The Sixth Joint Task Force of the European Society of Cardiology and Other Societies on Cardiovascular Disease Prevention in Clinical Practice. *Eur Heart J* 2016; 37: 2315–81.

10. Samayoa L, Grace SL, Gravely S, et al. Sex differences in cardiac rehabilitation enrolment: a meta-analysis. *Can J Cardiol* 2014; 30: 793–800.

11. Gravely S, Anand SS, Stewart DE, Grace SL. Effect of referral strategies on access to cardiac rehabilitation among women. *Eur J Prev Cardiol* 2014; 21: 1018–25.

12. Martin BJ, Arena R, Haykowsky M, et al. Cardiovascular fitness and mortality after contemporary cardiac rehabilitation. *Mayo Clin Proc* 2013; 88: 455–63.

13. Menezes AR, Lavie CJ, Forman DE, et al. Cardiac rehabilitation in the elderly. *Prog Cardiovasc Dis* 2014; 57: 152–9.

14. Buttery AK, Carr-White G, Martin FC, et al. Cardiac rehabilitation for heart failure. Do older people want to attend and are they referred? *Eur Geriatr Med* 2014; 5: 246–51.

15. McCorry NK, Corrigan M, Tully MA, et al. Perceptions of exercise among people who have not attended cardiac rehabilitation following myocardial infarction. *J Health Psychol* 2009; 14: 924–32.

16. Clark AM, King-Shier KM, Thompson DR, et al. A qualitative systematic review of influences on attendance at cardiac rehabilitation programs after referral. *Am Heart J* 2012; 164: 835–45

17. Jack BW, Chetty VK, Anthony D, et al. A reengineered hospital discharge program to decrease rehospitalization: a randomized trial. *Ann Intern Med* 2009; 150: 178–87.

18. Piepoli MF, Corrà U, Abreu A, et al. Challenges in secondary prevention of cardiovascular diseases: a review of the current practice. *Int J Cardiol* 2015; 180: 114–19.

19. Chow CK, Jolly S, Rao-Melacini P, et al. Association of diet, exercise, and smoking modification with risk of early cardiovascular events after acute coronary syndromes. *Circulation* 2010; 121: 750–8.

20. Kotseva K, De Backer G, De Bacquer D, et al. Lifestyle and impact on cardiovascular risk factor control in coronary patients across 27 countries: results from the European Society of Cardiology ESC-EORP EUROASPIRE V registry. *Eur J Prev Cardiol* 2019; 26: 824–35.

21. Cole JA, Smith SM, Hart N, Cupples ME. Do practitioners and friends support patients with coronary heart disease in lifestyle change? A qualitative study. *BMC Fam Pract* 2013; 14: 126.

22. National Institute for Health and Care Excellence. *Behaviour change: individual approaches. NICE Guideline PH49* January 2014. Available at: https://www.nice.org.uk/guidance/ph49

23. Naderi SH, Bestwick JP, Wald DS. Adherence to drugs that prevent cardiovascular disease: meta-analysis on 376,162 patients. *Am J Med* 2012; 125: 882–7.

24. Aubert RE, Yao J, Xia F, Garavaglia SB. Is there a relationship between early statin compliance and a reduction in healthcare utilization? *Am J Manag Care* 2010; 16: 459–66.

25. World Health Organization. *Adherence to Long-term Therapies: Evidence for Action.* Geneva: World Health Organization, 2003. Available at: http://who.int/chp/knowledge/publications/adherence_full_report.pdf (accessed 4 August 2019).

26. Nieuwlaat R, Wilczynski N, Navarro T, et al. Interventions for enhancing medication adherence. *Cochrane Database Syst Rev* 2014; (11): CD000011.

27. Gillebert TC, Brooks N, Fontes-Carvalho R, et al. ESC Core Curriculum for the General Cardiologist (2013). *Eur Heart J* 2013; 34: 2381–411.

28. OECD. *Health Usage Statistics. Length of Hospital Stay.* Available at: https://data.oecd.org/healthcare/length-of-hospital-stay.htm (accessed 5 August 2019).

29. Nieuwlaat R. Schwalm JD, Khatib R, Yusuf S. Why are we failing to implement effective therapies in cardiovascular disease? *Eur Heart J* 2013; 34: 1262–9.

30. Cupples ME, McKnight A. A five year follow-up study of patients at high cardiovascular risk who took part in a randomised controlled trial of health promotion. *BMJ* 1999; 319: 687–8.

31. BMA, NHS England. *Primary Care Strategy and NHS Contracts Group. 2019/20 General Medical Services (GMS) Contract Quality and Outcomes Framework (QOF). Guidance for GMS contract 2019/20 in England, April 2019.* available at https://www.england.nhs.uk/wp-content/uploads/2019/05/gms-contract-qof-guidance-april-2019.pdf (accessed 4 August 2019).

32. Piepoli MF, Binno S, Corrà U, et al. ExtraHF survey: the first European survey on implementation of exercise training in heart failure patients. *Eur J Heart Fail* 2015; 17(6): 631–8.

33. Hobbs FD, Jukema JW, Da Silva PM, et al. Barriers to cardiovascular disease risk scoring and primary prevention in Europe. *Q J Med* 2010; 103: 727–39.

34. West RR, Jones DA, Henderson AH. Rehabilitation After Myocardial Infarction Trial (RAMIT): multi-centre randomised controlled trial of comprehensive cardiac rehabilitation in patients following acute myocardial infarction. *Heart* 2012; 98(8): 637–44.

Further reading

Cupples ME, Cole JA, Hart ND, et al. Shared decision-making ('SHARE-D') for healthy behaviour change: feasibility study in general practice. *BJGP Open* 2018; 2: bjgpopen18X101517.

Heron N, Kee F, Donnelly M, et al. Behaviour change techniques in home-based cardiac rehabilitation: a systematic review. *Br J Gen Pract* 2016; 66: e747–57.

Kotseva K, De Backer G, De Bacquer D, Rydén L, Hoes A, Grobbee D, et al. Lifestyle and impact on cardiovascular risk factor control in coronary patients across 27 countries: results from the European Society of Cardiology ESC-EORP EUROASPIRE V registry. *Eur J Prev Cardiol* 2019; 26: 824–35.

Piepoli MF, Hoes AW, Agewall S, et al. European Guidelines on cardiovascular disease prevention in clinical practice. The Sixth Joint Task Force of the European Society of Cardiology and Other Societies on Cardiovascular Disease Prevention in Clinical Practice. *Eur Heart J* 2016; 37(29): 2315–81.

National Institute for Health and Care Excellence. *Behaviour change: individual approaches. NICE Guideline PH49* January 2014. Available at: https://www.nice.org.uk/guidance/ph49

Chapter 4

Human and material resources, structural, and organizational recommendations

Ana Abreu and Jean-Paul Schmid

Summary

Cardiac rehabilitation (CR) is recommended in the guidelines for patients with coronary artery disease (CAD) or heart failure (HF) because of its positive effect on morbidity and mortality. However, to ensure this, CR must be offered at a high standard, following recommended quality criteria. Human and material resources, as well as organizational aspects, are key factors for a successful CR programme. A multidisciplinary team is required to run a successful CR programme, with a cardiologist as director. Other specialized healthcare workers involved include exercise specialists, nutritionists, nurses, psychologists, and social workers, who must be available in the CR centre itself or on referral. The availability of infrastructural and material resources with dedicated spaces for exercise, education, consultation, and physical examination strongly depends on local conditions, but they must comply with the recommendations of a national working group or the EAPC/ESC.

Introduction

Quality criteria for CR concern not only the content of CR programmes (core components), but also human and material resources and organizational aspects, which have to satisfy specific quality criteria to ensure high standards of care in CR services [1]. These include the appropriateness of infrastructure and equipment and the qualifications required for the director/coordinator and the personnel who provide CR. Particular emphasis has to be placed on optimal medical treatment and management in order to ensure rapid response to medical emergencies that may occur during CR programme sessions.

Human resources and organizational issues

A multidisciplinary group, ideally consisting of a full-time dedicated team located in a designated physical space, is essential for the requirements of a CR programme [1]. However, most CR centres will not be able to have exclusive use of team members, but time dedicated to the CR programme must be assured and the team members must be able to cover all components of the CR programme. If some specific services, such as psychiatric consultation, are not available in the CR centre, patients may be sent to a referral centre. A range of schedules throughout the day should be offered to patients in order to increase CR uptake and overcome barriers to use.

The composition of the multidisciplinary team may vary depending on the recommendations in different countries, the availability of qualified personnel, the CR phase and the types of patient accepted for CR rehabilitation. Nevertheless, it is of utmost importance to respect the requirements of knowledge and competences to fulfil the needs for a recommended CR programme [1,2].

The following professionals should be available at the centre (indicated by an asterisk) or on a referral basis:

a) cardiologist (head or in charge of the CR Department)*

b) administrative personnel*

c) exercise specialists (physiotherapists, sports scientists)*

d) nutritionist*

e) nurses or other related healthcare professionals*

f) psychologist*

g) social worker

h) smoking cessation specialist

i) other physicians (diabetologist, psychiatrist, pneumologist, …).

The availability in some countries of national recommendations for professional certification and specific competences required for the personnel working in CR is a high-quality criterion. Whether or not team members have professional certification and specific competences in CR, they need continuous preparation and training. Therefore a description of the tasks and qualifications required for each team member should be available [1]:

a) required professional qualification

b) necessary education and training

c) responsibilities for delivering an appropriate standard of care

d) general duties (emergency procedures, liaison with other healthcare providers, basic skills in data collection and documentation, staff training, and performance reviews)

e) specific duties (patient counselling, interactive discussion groups, supervision of exercise sessions, referral procedure, programme management and coordination, discharge planning, and follow-up).

The programme coordinator/ director must be a cardiologist with advanced training in CR [1,2]. Training can take place via an internship or an externship (at least six months, depending on the number of patients using the centre), by participation in CR training courses, and by online learning tools to ascertain his/her CR competences (defined by EAPC/ESC). The minimal standards of training can be defined by the national working group/association/society on CR as well as EAPC/ESC.

In addition to his/her clinical expertise, the programme director should have organizational experience. He/she is responsible for the organization of the programme (effectiveness and safety) and the supervision of the CR team. His/her main roles are to guarantee that:

a) all team members have the necessary qualifications and certifications, are carrying out their tasks satisfactorily, and are trained in basic life support

b) the patient's progress during the programme is followed regularly

c) the initially defined aims are achieved

d) patient care has the recommended quality

e) legislation is implemented

f) a periodic report on the activities of CR or outcome measures is produced

g) risk to the patient is minimized by correct supervision and monitoring as needed.

Cardiologists should evaluate the patient before starting the exercise programme, identify and manage risk factors (RFs), confirm adherence to therapy, stratify cardiac risk, and prescribe exercise. The prescription of aerobic exercise intensity should be individually determined, based on the results of the initial clinical assessment and an exercise stress test (EST) supervised by a cardiologist with experience in exercise [1–3].

During the exercise sessions exercise specialists implement the prescribed exercise intensity, adapted to the patient's functional status, and inform the cardiologist on exercise progression (and how the patient perceives exercise) and any medical problems. They coordinate exercise training and are responsible for its content and adaptation of exercise intensity. As a general rule, one exercise specialist should supervise five to ten low- or intermediate-risk patients in a session. The ratio may be lower for high-risk patients. For safety, it is mandatory that another healthcare professional, in addition to the exercise specialist, is present in the exercise room. If the cardiologist is not in the room, he/she needs to be contactable or, if he/she is not available, a medical back-up must be on hand to ensure a rapid intervention in the case of complications or an emergency [3].

Nutritionists evaluate the patient's nutritional status and are responsible for teaching the principles of a healthy heart diet. They advise on weight modification and RF management when necessary (e.g. in the case of diabetes mellitus).

Psychologists are responsible for interpreting screening tools for psychosocial RFs, in particularly depression and anxiety, but also post-traumatic stress disorder. They should be able to provide or mediate appropriate management when needed. Cognitive behavioural therapy and relaxation techniques may be most useful.

Nurses in particular, but also cardiologists, nutritionists, and exercise specialists, have an important role in education regarding diet, physical activity (PA), RF control including smoking, and advice on exercise, driving, work, and sexual activity.

If available, social workers are important, in particular in phases I and II. They can help with a variety of problems that occur after an acute cardiac event, including social (re-)integration, finances, and problems with insurance. Vocational counselling should be addressed in close collaboration with the cardiologist.

It is important to produce an organizational chart showing the number of people in each professional discipline in the team, the number of permanent or temporary consultants, and the staff–patient ratio. While more than one member of the team can share more than one task, some tasks require specific skills and training and should be performed by a specially designated health professional.

Regular meetings (every week or two weeks) are important to facilitate communication between team members and to provide opportunities to discuss complex clinical cases.

Electronic files for CR consultations and examinations are desirable. All clinical data should be digitally stored in a specific CR database from which clinical information can be extracted and sent to a national database when needed.

Organizational aspects, infrastructural and material resources

Patients eligible for a CR programme

The availability of a referral path to CR, ideally an automatic process to ensure that all eligible patients are directed to the CR programme, and close communication with the referring physicians are crucial to assure a constant enrolment of patients in the programme.

Indications for CR are:

a) condition after an ACS or chronic CAD with or without CABG or PCI
b) stable CAD with multiple RFs
c) diffuse CAD or incompletely revascularized CAD (complete revascularization not possible) with ischaemia
d) stable HF
e) pulmonary hypertension
f) congenital heart disease which has been surgically corrected
g) condition after implantation of an assist device or heart transplantation
h) condition after implantation of a resynchronization device, defibrillator, or pacemaker
i) condition after valve surgery or percutaneous implantation of prosthetic valves or clips
j) condition after surgery on the aorta.

Objectives

A well-designed multidisciplinary CR programme should have the following aims:

a) Improvement of CV function, functional capacity, muscular strength, balance, and flexibility by individualizing the exercise programme in terms of intensity, duration, frequency, modality, and type of PA according to the patient's ability and interest.

b) Detection and treatment of arrhythmias, haemodynamic changes, and electrocardiographic changes during and outside the exercise sessions.

c) Optimization of pharmacological therapy and promotion of medication adherence.

d) Identification and control of RFs.

e) Educating the patient on how to exercise and remain active in the long term.

f) Working with the patients and their close family or caregivers to help them adopting a healthier lifestyle including:

　(i) education on nutrition

　(ii) education on CV disease, RFs and medication.

g) Evaluation and improvement of the patient's psychological condition.

h) Promotion of the patient's autonomy and empowerment.

i) Advising on return to work, travelling, driving, sexual activity, and physical activity

Infrastructural and material requirements

Ideally, facilities should include [1–3]:

a) gymnasium

b) dressing-room (ideally with a shower)

c) waiting room

d) education room (which can be the exercise room).

The CR programme should offer endurance activities and strength training using material adapted to the needs of the target population. Flexibility, coordination, and balance training, which are particularly useful in older patients, should also be available.

At a minimum, the following equipment should be available:

a) treadmills and cycle ergometers

b) elastic bands and equipment for weight training

c) sphygmomanometer, chronometer, and digital oximeter

d) electrocardiogram (ECG) monitoring

e) cardiorespiratory resuscitation equipment

When to begin

Phase I

Phase I, the hospital phase, begins as soon as the patient stabilizes after the acute event (usually after 24-48 hours), as determined by the intensive care unit physician.

Early intervention during the hospital stay includes early mobilization and prevention of complications secondary to immobilization, as well as early screening for RF, education at discharge, and referral for phase II [2].

Phase II

The patient should start phase II, early ambulatory, as soon as possible, preferably within two weeks after discharge or, for non-hospitalized patients, after diagnosis. Early start of CR increases compliance and enables the patient to profit from the positive effects of exercise training on myocardial remodelling after an acute event.

The initial assessment and CV risk stratification (low, intermediate, or high) is performed by the programme's cardiologist. This stratification is based mainly on symptom severity, degree of left ventricular dysfunction, functional capacity, and the presence of residual ischaemia or arrhythmias [4].

Complementary examinations required for this assessment include exercise testing (in HF patients preferably cardiopulmonary exercise testing (CPET) with respiratory gas analysis), echocardiography (plus other imaging methods if necessary), and Holter monitoring (mainly for patients with arrhythmias).

Exercise testing is also essential for prescription of aerobic exercise intensity and must be performed in all cases where patients are able to perform an EST. For those unable to perform such a test, the six-minute walk test is an alternative for documentation of exercise performance and improvements. However, it is not suitable for exercise prescription or analysis of haemodynamic response to exercise, including the occurrence of arrhythmias.

At the end of a phase II CR programme the patient should be reassessed (clinical status, functional status, cardiac function, laboratory analysis, HRQoL, nutritional status, psychological status, etc.) in order to document the progress achieved during the programme and to quantify the benefits.

A CR report including the disease, the progress achieved in functional, psychological, nutritional, RF control, remaining problems, the goals still to achieve, continuing medication, specific advice for PA, diet, and work should be prepared by the cardiologist. This report is given to the patient to deliver to the GP and the assistant cardiologist in phase III CR.

Phase III

After completing phase II, the patient should be encouraged to continue regular long-term PA. A phase III should be offered if available (generally in a community-based centre or as a home-based programme). The patient can continue regular exercise under the instruction of a physical therapist, usually supervised by a cardiologist, and maintain nutritional and psychological support.

Hybrid CR (HBCR) (part of the programme in a centre, part at home) with supervision and/or monitoring at distance (when necessary) is available in some countries[5]. It is a good alternative for patients who cannot attend phase III CR because of difficulties, such as travel distance or work schedule.

Follow-up of patients who have performed a CR phase II programme by nurses or other team members is desirable and can be performed via periodical consultations or also phone or mail. These contacts can be used to monitor and coach patients with respect to the long-term continuation of healthy life habits.

Conclusion

CR programmes need to satisfy minimum quality standards, including human, infrastructural, and material resources. The programme should be led a cardiologist who is responsible for its organization, including all the requirements of a multidisciplinary secondary prevention programme. Furthermore, the programme should comply with the recommendations of the EAPC/ESC guidelines and the recommendations of the National Society of Cardiology or the corresponding Working Group or Association of Cardiac Rehabilitation.

CR should be embedded in a continuous patient process, starting with admission to hospital during the acute phase, followed by the specialized care during phase II rehabilitation, and continuing for life in a phase III centre or in a home-based or hybrid programme, thus ensuring the continuation of long-term healthy habits.

References

1. Piepoli M, Corrá U, Adamapoulos S., et al. Secondary prevention in the clinical management of patients with cardiovascular diseases. Core components, standards and outcome measures for referral and deliver. *Eur J Prev Cardiol* 2014; 21: 664–81.

2. Abreu A, Frederix I, Dendale P, et al. Standardization and quality improvement of secondary prevention through cardiovascular rehabilitation programmes in Europe: The avenue towards EAPC accreditation programme: A position statement of the Secondary Prevention and Rehabilitation Section of the European Association of Preventive Cardiology (EAPC). *Eur J Prev Cardiol* 2020, https://doi.org/10.1177/2047487320924912.

3. Abreu A, Mendes M, Dores H, et al. Mandatory criteria for cardiac rehabilitation programs: 2018 guidelines from the Portuguese Society of Cardiology. *Rev Port Cardiol* 2018; 37: 363–73.

4. França da Silva AK, Barbosa MPC, Bernardo AFBB, et al. Cardiac risk stratification in cardiac rehabilitation programs: a review of protocols. *Rev Bras Cir Cardiovasc* 2014; 29(2): 255–65.

5. Imran H, Baig M, Ergou S, et al. Home-based cardiac rehabilitation alone and hybrid with center-based cardiac rehabilitation in heart failure: a systematic review and meta-analysis. *J Am Heart Assoc* 2019; 8: e012779.

Further reading

Ambrosetti M, Abreu A, Corrà U, et al. Secondary prevention through comprehensive cardiovascular rehabilitation: from knowledge to implementation. 2020 update. A position paper from the Secondary Prevention and Rehabilitation Section of the European Association of Preventive Cardiology. *Eur J Prev Cardiol* 2020, https://doi.org/10.1177/2047487320913379.

Cowie A, Buckley J, Doherty P, et al. Standards and core components for cardiovascular disease prevention and rehabilitation. *Heart* 2019; 105: 510–15.

Chapter 5

Recovering from acute heart events

Ugo Corrà and Jean-Paul Schmid

Summary

Despite extraordinary advances in pharmacological and interventional therapies, cardiac rehabilitation (CR) and secondary prevention programmes have maintained a class I indication with level of evidence A in patients after acute coronary syndrome (ACS) and a class I recommendation with level of evidence B in patients after surgical revascularization and with chronic ischaemic heart disease (IHD). In post-acute or chronic heart failure (New York Heart Association (NYHA) class II–III, both with reduced or preserved ejection fraction (EF)), CR has a class I recommendation with level of evidence A. In patients with recent valvular heart surgery, there is an important indication for CR intervention early after surgery. Once admitted to CR, patients should have their clinical status assessed or reviewed before starting any activities, particularly exercise training. Assessment should cover medical history, personal goals and preferences, physical parameters, disease-specific status, disease management, psychosocial health, risk factors (RFs), functional exercise capacity, health-related quality of life (HRQoL), and the impact of physical deconditioning of comorbidities. Previous exercise levels, aids used, goals, and residual exercise capacity/function should also be considered. If patients are not clinically stable, CR interventions should be deferred. However, if patients are stable, intervention should be started as soon as possible after an acute cardiac event after appropriate functional assessment.

35

Introduction

Experiencing a heart attack is very stressful, and patients need support to live with a new heart condition, staying as healthy as possible and reducing the risk of recurrence. The primary goal of CR is to reduce the risk of a future cardiac event by stabilizing, slowing, or even reversing the progression of cardiovascular disease (CVD) [1,2].

Cardiac rehabilitation after acute heart events

The intervention (CR) generally takes place in three phases [3]. Phase I, during acute hospital stay, includes:

a) reassurance
b) supportive counselling
c) early mobilization (EM)
d) prevention of complications secondary to immobilization
e) discharge planning and referral to outpatient rehabilitation.

Phase II promotes and delivers preventive and rehabilitative services, including risk stratification and promotion of long-term adherence:

a) optimization of medical therapy to relieve symptoms (breathlessness or angina), promote recovery of cardiac function, and avoid negative remodelling
b) starting physical exercise and improving exercise capacity
c) restoring self-confidence, treating anxiety and depression, and preparing to resume daily activities, social functioning, and professional reintegration
d) controlling CV RFs (quit all forms of smoking, have a healthy diet, implement regular physical activity (PA), and adhere to preventive medications)
e) home-based programmes are an alternative to centre-based programmes and can be delivered in the patient's home, supported by educational materials, periodic visits to the CR centre, and contacts with the CR team.

Phase III is the long-term (lifelong) promotion of PA and maintenance of a healthy lifestyle (smoking cessation, healthy nutrition, RF control, psychological equilibrium), mostly with some involvement of and support from outpatient CR.

In some countries, CR services are available as dedicated inpatient programmes. These are particularly suitable for high-risk patients, such as the following:

a) patients with persistent clinical instability because of complications after an acute event or intervention (pleural or pericardial effusion, arrhythmias, etc.)
b) patients with advanced heart failure (HF)
c) after heart transplantation or implantation of a ventricular assist device (VAD)
d) frail patients or patients with severe or multiple comorbidities [2].

Despite extraordinary advances in pharmacological and interventional therapies, CR has maintained a class I indication with level of evidence A in patients after ACS and a class I recommendation with level of evidence B in patients after surgical revascularization and those with chronic IHD [3]. The guidelines also report a class I recommendation with level of evidence A for CR in post-acute or chronic HF (NYHA class II–III, both with reduced or preserved EF) [1–4]. In addition, there is a strong indication for CR intervention early after valvular heart surgery [3].

Thus, almost all CVD patients should be referred to CR after recovery from an acute event [4], but there is marked delay in referral (about a week to four months). Unfortunately, activities during this period are not mentioned. It should be noted that timely access to CR programmes can provide reassurance to patients and family members, ensure prompt receipt of education and intervention for RFs that may or may not be provided before hospital discharge, and encourage earlier adoption of behaviours promoting heart health [5]. Furthermore, delayed access to CR may negatively affect the patient's perception of requirements. Accordingly, the Canadian Cardiovascular Society Access to Care Working Group on Rehabilitation has published guidelines on waiting times. It defines a waiting time between referral and CR between 0 and 30 days as 'preferable', and between 7 and 60 days as 'acceptable' [6]. Times from post-discharge referral to the start of a CR programme for CAD patients was equal to or less than the national median of England (33 days), Northern Ireland (40 days), or Wales (26 days). The same was true after heart surgery (CABG): England 46 days, Northern Ireland 52 days, and Wales 42 days [7]. Patients with early appointments for CR interventions showed significantly improved attendance and safety [8].

Once admitted to in- or outpatient CR, all CVD patients should have their clinical status carefully assessed or reviewed before starting activities, particularly exercise programmes [9]. The following evaluations may be considered:

a) resting 12-lead electrocardiogram
b) resting echocardiography
c) exercise stress testing, with or without gas exchange monitoring (depending on the patient's condition and residual LV function); if patients are unable to perform a maximal stress test, a six-minute walk test may be an alternative
d) 24 h (Holter) or longer electrocardiographic monitoring if cardiac arrhythmias are suspected [2].

Assessment should also cover medical history, personal goals and preferences, physical parameters, disease-specific status, disease management, psychosocial health, RFs, functional exercise capacity, HRQoL, and the impact of comorbidities on decreased physical capacity [2,3]. Moreover, assessment should include previous exercise levels, aids used, goals, and residual exercise capacity/function. This is an essential part of tailoring a programme to the requirements of the patient and setting goals (Box 5.1). A comprehensive, multidisciplinary, and holistic approach is a prerequisite for starting a CR programme [3,9].

There are some contraindications to CR attendance, particularly regarding the uptake of physical exercise in the context of medically unstable conditions [10]. Participation in EM or exercise testing (ET) by patients with known heart disease poses a number of clinical and ethical questions, including determining the most appropriate physical activities in which patients may safely be engaged [11]. Identification of a heart disease, or the incidence of a cardiac event, is usually associated with prudent advice for patients to reduce (or leave) intensive ET, justified by clinical concern for the increased cardiac risk associated with exercise. Healthcare professionals are often faced with the dilemma of whether exercise-based CR should be prescribed, knowing that EM or ET is not advisable for some medical conditions. Thus, participation in exercise-based CR depends on appropriate clinical and functional assessment. Since exercise is medically prescribed and supervised, the risks should be low, and most CVD patients are eligible to participate. CR providers tailor the ET programme to the medical needs of individual patients, and any recommendation for EM and/or ET should be based on the pathology of the patient's condition, the

- Demographic characteristics: age, gender, race.
- Social situation: family, social network, details of any community services being received, whether the person identifies with a particular cultural background, hobbies/interests, relevant financial information, and usual transport arrangements (e.g. driving, community transport, family members).
- Recent and previous cardiac events: detailed clinical description.
- Precipitating causes (if present): are they controlled by treatment or other lifestyle measures?
- Concomitant disease (if present): is it active and potentially limiting exercise capacity?
- Results of clinical and imaging examinations in the acute state and description of patient's trajectory (improvement, stability, and deterioration).
- Prescribed cardioprotective therapies, including medication and implantable devices.
- Outcome of cardiac event (i.e. left ventricular dysfunction, persistent arrhythmias, myocardial ischaemia, haemodynamic instability, symptom perseverance, etc.), i.e. risk stratification after the acute phase.
- Clinical and (new) imaging examinations before attending CR programmes.
- Residual physical capabilities and needs after an acute cardiac event or worsening of chronic CVD: mobility and transfers, level of independence with activities of daily living, information on the need for any aids/equipment/modifications and/or physical assistance.
- Psychosocial and cognitive factors.
- Identify any pain that could impact on activity, quality of life, or capacity to self-manage.
- Identify the patient's main problems, set personalized goals, and determine how the goals will be achieved (self-management) in collaboration with the patient.
- Prescribe an individualized exercise programme which is safe and effective.
- Assessment of fitness/functional capacity before cardiac event (or worsening of chronic CVD).

individual's response to exercise (including heart rate, blood pressure, symptoms, and perceived exertion), and functional measurements made during ET [11].

Conclusion

There is good scientific evidence that CR improves prognosis and it is strongly recommended for all CVD patients. However, if patients are not clinically and functionally stable, CR interventions should be deferred. When a stable clinical condition is established and after appropriate functional assessment, in- or outpatient CR should be started as soon as possible after an acute cardiac event or intervention.

References

1. Balady GJ, Ades PA, Bittner VA, et al. Referral, enrollment, and delivery of cardiac rehabilitation/secondary prevention programs at clinical centers and beyond: a presidential advisory from the American Heart Association. *Circulation* 2011; 124: 2951–60.
2. Piepoli MF, Corrà U, Benzer W, et al. Secondary prevention through cardiac rehabilitation: from knowledge to implementation. A position paper from the Cardiac Rehabilitation Section of the

European Association of Cardiovascular Prevention and Rehabilitation. *Eur J Cardiovasc Prev Rehabil* 2010; 17: 1–17.

3. Piepoli M, Corrà U, Adamopoulos S, et al. Secondary prevention in the clinical management of patients with cardiovascular diseases. Core components, standards and outcome measures for referral and delivery. *Eur J Prev Cardiol* 2014; 21: 664–8.

4. Piepoli MF, Hoes AW, Agewall S, et al. 2016 European Guidelines on cardiovascular disease prevention in clinical practice. *Eur Heart J* 2016; 37: 2315–61.

5. Collins CL, Suskin N, Aggarwall S, Grace SL Cardiac rehabilitation wait times and relation to patient outcomes. *Eur J Phys Rehabil Med* 2014; 51: 301–9.

6. Dafoe W, Arthur H, Stokes H, et al. Universal access: but when? Treating the right patient at the right time. Access to cardiac rehabilitation. *Can J Cardiol* 2006; 22: 905–11.

7. British Association for Cardiovascular Prevention and Rehabilitation (BACPR). *The BACPR Standards and Core Components for Cardiovascular Disease Prevention and Rehabilitation.* London: British Cardiovascular Society, 2017. Available at http://www.bacpr.com/resources/AC6_BACPRStandards&CoreComponents2017.pdf

8. Pack QR, Mansour M, Barboza JS, et al. An early appointment to outpatient cardiac rehabilitation at hospital discharge improves attendance at orientation. A randomized, single-blind, controlled trial. *Circulation* 2013; 127: 349–55.

9. Turk-Adawi K, Oldridge N, Tarima SS, et al. Cardiac rehabilitation patient and organizational factors: what keeps patients in programs? *J Am Heart Assoc* 2013; 2: e000418.

10. Piepoli M, Corrà U, Abreu A, et al. Challenges in secondary prevention of cardiovascular diseases: a review of the current practice. *Int J Cardiol* 2015; 180: 114–19.

11. Pavy B, Iliou MC, Meurin P, et al. Safety of exercise training for cardiac patients: results of the French registry of complications during cardiac rehabilitation. *Arch Intern Med* 2006; 166: 2329–34.

Further reading

Ji H, Fang L, Yuan L, Zhang Q. Effects of exercise-based cardiac rehabilitation in patients with acute coronary syndrome: a meta-analysis. *Med Sci Monit* 2019; 25: 5015–27

Mampuya WM. Cardiac rehabilitation past, present and future; an overview. *Cardiovasc Diagn Ther* 2012; 2: 38–49

Rauch B, Avos CH, Doherty P, et al. The prognostic effect of cardiac rehabilitation in the era of acute revascularization and statin therapy: a systematic review and meta-analysis of randomized and non-randomized studies—The Cardiac Rehabilitation Outcome Study (CROS). *Eur J Prev Cardiol* 2016: 23; 1914–19.

Chapter 6

Early assessment and risk stratification

Marie Christine Iliou and Catherine Monpere

Summary

A pre-participation medical assessment before cardiac rehabilitation (CR) is mandatory in order to deliver a safe programme tailored to the individual patient. This initial evaluation also aims to increase patient adherence and the efficiency of the programme. The entry assessment includes the following components: history, global patient evaluation including clinical questionnaires, physical examination, laboratory analysis, and non-invasive cardiovascular testing. Following this assessment, a risk stratification should be performed to determine the appropriate CR modalities.

Introduction

The core components required for a CR programme should be comprehensively evaluated [1]. Clinical, physical, biological, and non-invasive tests, and also psychosocial assessments, are required in order to determine the individual risk profile and to deliver the best tailored management. This means that not only cardiologists but also other healthcare professionals (i.e. nurses, physiotherapists, psychologists, nutritionists, etc.) must participate in this evaluation [2].

Early assessment

Clinical

History and interview
The index event diagnosis must be clearly recorded. Currently, CR is indicated in a large variety of diagnoses: coronary artery disease at different stages (acute coronary syndrome, percutaneous coronary intervention, stable angina), heart failure (HF) patients (reduced and preserved ejection fraction, pre- and post-transplant), postoperative (coronary artery bypass grafting (CABG), valvular, aorta), congenital heart diseases, cardiac devices including pacemakers (PMs), cardiac resynchronization therapy (CRT), implantable cardioverter–defibrillator (ICD), left-ventricular assist device (LVAD), and peripheral artery disease (PAD). Frequently, several diagnoses

are associated in one patient (e.g. ischaemic cardiomyopathy due to a large myocardial infarction (MI), HF patients wearing an implantable device, or the patient's condition after CABG and PAD) which increases the severity of the patient's condition.

Usually, patients are referred to CR after an acute event, and the evolution during the acute phase is one of the criteria determining the risk profile and therefore may modify the CR modalities prescribed.

The symptoms declared by the patients must be specified and reported (angina, dyspnoea, palpitations, fatigue) using NYHA functional class for dyspnoea and the Canadian Cardiovascular Society (CCS) class for angina.

According to the ESC guidelines on prevention, all cardiovascular risk factors (CV RFs) should be assessed: arterial hypertension, diabetes mellitus (DM), overweight/obesity, sedentary habits/inactivity, smoking, dyslipidaemia, positive family history, and other non-classic RFs [3].

Among the comorbidities and disabilities, chronic obstructive pulmonary disease (COPD), renal failure, anemia, orthopaedic problems, neurological problems, frailty, and sleep apnoeas must be considered.

The medical treatment regimen deserves particular attention: knowledge of drugs, good tolerance, and adherence are required. Similarly, drug optimization and titration should be implemented during the CR programme in collaboration with the attending physicians.

If the patient benefits from a cardiac implanted electronic device (PM, ICD), its type, characteristics, mode of intervention, and thresholds must be recorded.

The psychological evaluation is performed through different scales: a simple interview or questionnaires, such as the Hospital Anxiety Depression Scale (HADS) or the Patient Health Questionnaire (PHQ) [4]. HRQoL evaluation can be collected using an outcome tool such as the HeartQoL questionnaire for patients with chronic ischaemic disease or the Kansas City Questionnaire or the Minnesota Living with Heart Failure Questionnaire for patients with HF. Cognitive evaluation is only be needed for patients with suspicion of dementia.

Patients' previous lifestyle behaviours (domestic, occupational, and recreational habits), motivation, knowledge, and expectations (self-confidence, readiness to change) must be noted for educational purposes. Asking about vocational status is important for adapting counselling and the objectives of CR and for determining the patient's ability to work.

Physical examination

A general physical examination must be performed including vital signs (resting heart rate (HR) and blood pressure (BP)), weight, body mass index (BMI), waist circumference, general health status, cardiac and lung auscultation, peripheral pulses, and ankle-brachial index. This examination must be personalized according to the main diagnoses and comorbidities (signs of congestion, signs of cachexia, reduced muscle mass, sternotomy scar evaluation, pleural effusion).

Tests

1. A resting ECG allows determination of rhythm, HR, conduction disturbances, signs of ischaemia, and alterations in repolarization.

2. Laboratory testing has to be adjusted to the specific diagnosis, but routine biochemical assays may include a full blood count, electrolytes, renal and liver function, fasting blood glucose and/or HbA1c, blood lipids (total cholesterol, low- and high-density lipoprotein cholesterol (LDL-C, HDL-C, and triglycerides), and brain natriuretic peptide (BNP/NTpro-BNP).

3. Resting 2D-Doppler echocardiography is essential to determine left ventricular ejection fraction (LVEF), left ventricle volumes, right ventricular function and volume, valvular abnormalities, presence of an effusion, intraventricular thrombus, left ventricular filling pressure, and pulmonary arterial pressure.

4. If necessary, arrhythmias (ventricular tachyarrhythmias, atrial fibrillation) can also be assessed by 24-hour ambulatory ECG monitoring and/or ECG telemetry.

5. In selected cases, sleep tests may be needed to screen for the occurrence of nocturnal breathing disorders.

6. Physical fitness evaluation.
   • Exercise stress testing (EST): ECG-monitored symptom-limited exercise testing on either a cyclo-ergometer or a treadmill. Cardiopulmonary exercise testing (CPET) is also used, and is highly recommended for patients with HF, transplants, or congenital heart disease. The EST protocol (i.e. maximal or sub-maximal) should be adapted to the patient's condition. If EST is not feasible, a six-minute walk test or a shuttle walk test should be considered. This evaluation is essential not only for the prognosis, but also to prescribe the appropriate exercise training and to optimize the drug regimen. The minimum data that must be recorded are test duration, workload, and HR with the percentage of the predicted maximal value, BP profile during exercise and recovery, occurrence of ischaemia and arrhythmias, and the reason for terminating the test.
   • Muscular strength can be tested using various methods: isometric or dynamic strength using the one or ten repetition maximum (1-RM or 10-RM) or dynamometer testing for large muscle groups in the upper and lower limbs and for the dorsal and gluteus muscular groups. Measurement of maximal inspiratory pressure is widely accepted for respiratory musculature testing.
   • In general, and particularly for COPD, spirometry must be performed.

A check list is presented in (Table 6.1).

Risk profile

According to the European guidelines, all patients after a CV event should be considered to be at very high risk. However, additional risk stratification must be performed for these patients to personalize the CR programme: inpatient or outpatient programme, CV supervision modality, safety issues, and patient counselling/education. In general, the exercise-related risk during CR is low, but strict supervision should be considered if necessary.

Table 6.1 Check list for assessment before CR			
Evaluation	Tasks/core components	Tools	Other components
Demographics	Age, gender, race		
Index event	History of patient Acute event: date, evolution	Referral letter or hospital discharge report and interview	
Medical treatment	Control of tolerance and compliance	Drug prescription	
Residual symptoms	Angina, palpitations, dyspnoea, fatigue	Interview, NYHA class and CCS	
CV risk factors	History, behaviours Assessments	Interview about known CV risk, smoking, physical activity, and nutrition Blood testing: blood count, cholesterol, HDL, LDL, triglycerides, glycaemia, Hb1Ac	BNP/NTproBNP C-reactive protein
Clinical examination	Global physical health CV examination	Vital signs: HR, BP, waist, BMI	Other specific tests: congestion, cachexia, scar evaluation, ...
Comorbidities	History, clinical evaluation of: renal, pulmonary, liver diseases rheumatology, osteo-articular, neurology limitations Frailty	Interview, referral letter, reports and physical examination Renal, liver function (blood testing), chest X-ray Physical examination Edmonton frailty scale, CSHA frailty scale	
Cardiiovascular function	Non- invasive testing	Resting ECG Cardiac echo-Doppler Holter ECG/ telemetry Exercise test (CPET)	Stress-echo MRI Sleep apnoea screening, ABI
Exercise capacity	Exercise testing	Symptom- limited ECG exercise test/ CPET (if possible for all, recommended for HF)	6 min walk test, shuttle test
Psychological	Stress Anxiety and depression Quality of life	Stress scale HAD SF30, Mc New QOL Kansas City or Minessota (HF patients)	
Social	Workplace Social conditions Educational level	Intensity demand Psychological burden Interview	Ainsworth compendium Family, social network, cultural background, income and transport facilities

The risk classification originally proposed by Haskell is used (Box 6.1) [5]. Other parameters such as age, gender, CV RFs, and psychosocial status must also be considered as risk modifiers. Application of this classification will result in different types of management:

- unstable patients at very high risk needing 24-hour supervision should initially receive residential CR
- high-risk patients need close monitoring and supervision during ET sessions
- low-risk patients may be eligible for home-based programmes.

Box 6.1 Proposed risk stratification at CR entry

High risk

- Patients with severe *in-hospital* complications.
- Patients with persistent clinical instability, ischaemia or arrhythmias after the acute event.
- Serious concomitant diseases at high risk of cardiovascular events.
- Patients with advanced congestive heart failure (NYHA class III and IV), and/or severe ventricular dysfunction, and/or needing mechanical support.
- Patients after a recent heart transplant.
- Patients discharged very early after the acute event (<1–2 weeks depending on the index event) even if uncomplicated, and particularly if they are older, female, frail, or at higher risk of progression of CVD.
- Exercise performance <4 METs.
- Survivors after sudden death.
- Social deprivation, low income.
- Depression.

Low risk

- Long delay (>1–2 months) after uncomplicated acute event.
- Stable (asymptomatic, e.g. CCS = 0, NHYA = 1), uncomplicated patient.
- Exercise capacity >6 METs or >50% of predicted values.
- No residual ischaemia.
- No ventricular dysfunction.
- No severe arrhythmias.
- No uncontrolled hypertension.
- Absence of comorbidities.
- No cardiac implanted electronic devices.
- Autonomy without psychosocial risk.

  All other patients should be considered at intermediate risk.

Source data from Fletcher GF, Ades PA, Kligfield P, et al. American Heart Association Exercise, Cardiac Rehabilitation, and Prevention Committee of the Council on Clinical Cardiology, Council on Nutrition, Physical Activity and Metabolism, Council on Cardiovascular and Stroke Nursing, and Council on Epidemiology and Prevention. Exercise standards for testing and training: a scientific statement from the American Heart Association. *Circulation* 2013;128(8):873-934.

Box 6.2 Contraindications to exercise testing and/or training

Absolute

- STEMI/non STEMI <2 days or unstable angina not previously stabilized.
- Severe and uncontrolled cardiac arrhythmias.
- Uncontrolled symptomatic heart failure.
- Severe and symptomatic obstruction to ventricular outflow.
- Acute deep vein thrombosis with or without pulmonary embolism.
- Acute myocarditis, pericarditis, or endocarditis.
- Acute aortic dissection.
- Intra-cardiac thrombus with high risk of embolism.
- Inability to exercise adequately or patient refusal.
- Significant pericardial effusion.

Relative / temporary (at discretion of cardiologist)

- Significant left main artery stenosis.
- Ventricular aneurysm.
- Supraventricular tachycardia with uncontrolled ventricular rate.
- Recent stroke or transient ischaemic attack.
- Uncorrected medical condition (marked anaemia, electrolyte imbalance).
- Severe arterial hypertension (resting BP >200/100).
- Hypertrophic cardiomyopathy with outflow tract obstruction at rest.
- Lack of patient cooperation.

STEMI, ST elevation myocardial infarction

Reproduced from Marcadet DM, Pavy B, Bosser G, et al. French Society of Cardiology guidelines on exercise tests (part 1): Methods and interpretation. *Arch Cardiovasc Dis* 2018;111(12):782-790. doi:10.1016/j.acvd.2018.05.005 with permission from Elsevier.

Conclusion

Thorough assessment of patients entering a CR programme is necessary, including all aspects of a multidisciplinary programme. This enables the programme to be personalized as much as possible, stratifying risk and ruling out contraindications (Box 6.2).

References

1. Piepoli M, Corrà U, Benzer W, et al. Secondary prevention through cardiac rehabilitation: from knowledge to implementation. *Eur J Cardiovasc Prev Rehabil* 2010; 17: 1–17.
2. Fattirolli F, Bettinardi O, Angelino E, et al. What constitutes the 'minimal care' interventions of the nurse, physiotherapist, dietician and psychologist in cardiovascular rehabilitation and

secondary prevention. A position paper from the Italian Association for Cardiovascular Prevention, Rehabilitation and Epidemiology. *Eur J Prev Cardiol* 2018; 25: 1799–1810

3. Piepoli M, Corrà U, Adamopoulos S, et al. Secondary prevention in the clinical management of patients with cardiovascular diseases. Core components, standards and outcome measures for referral and delivery. *Eur J Prev Cardiol* 2014; 21: 664–81.

4. van Engen-Verheul M, Kemps H, de Keizer N, et al. Revision of the Dutch clinical algorithm for assessing patients needs in cardiac rehabilitation based on identified implementation problems. *Eur J Prev Cardiol* 2011; 19: 504–14.

5. Marcadet D, Pavy B, Bosser G, et al. French Society of Cardiology guidelines on exercise test (part1). *Arch Cardiovasc Dis* 2018; 111: 782–90.

Further reading

Price K, Gordon B, Bird S, Benson A. A review of guidelines for cardiac rehabilitation exercise programmes. Is there an international consensus? *Eur J Prev Cardiol* 2016; 23: 1715–33.

Chapter 7

Modalities of physical activity and exercise in the management of cardiovascular health in individuals with cardiovascular risk factors

Dominique Hansen and Martin Halle

Summary

Physical activity (PA) and exercise training (ET) are highly effective in the prevention of cardiovascular disease (CVD) via improvement of cardiovascular risk factors (CV RFs), such as blood pressure (BP), lipid profile, glycaemic control, body fat mass, and inflammation. In the first part of this chapter, we describe the currently observed effects of PA and exercise intervention on these RFs. In the second part, we explain which exercise modalities should be selected to optimize these CVD RFs, especially for those patients with multiple CVD RFs.

49

Introduction

When individuals are physically active or participate in an ET intervention, the likelihood of suffering from major CVD is reduced by approximately 25% (hazard ratio 0.69–0.82, when comparing <150 min exercise per week versus >750 min exercise per week) [1]. Moreover, habitual PA is associated with a lower all-cause mortality as observed in 36,383 middle-aged and older adults with hazard ratios for mortality over a 5.8 year follow-up decreasing from 1.0 in the low activity quartile (reference group) to 0.48 (95% CI 0.43–0.54) in the second quartile, 0.34 (95% CI 0.26–0.45) in the third quartile, and to 0.27 (95% CI 0.23–0.32) in the most active quartile [2]. In addition to the major effects on CVD, a high PA level is also related to a lower incidence of cancer, osteoporosis, and dementia.

Therefore current guidelines strongly recommend PA and ET (class 1A) in the primary prevention of CVD as a key factor for healthy ageing and avoidance of premature death [3]. Despite this evidence, exercise is insufficiently prescribed in routine practice. Therefore it is important for clinicians (1) to understand the efficacy of PA or ET in improving CVD RFs and (2) how to prescribe exercise for maximal improvement in CVD risk profiles.

First, we will provide an overview of the effects of PA and ET on different CVD RFs, and secondly we focus on how to prescribe exercise for patients with different combinations of CVD RFs.

Effects of physical activity and exercise training on CVD risk factors

The latest evidence shows that PA and ET have significant positive impact on CVD RFs (Table 7.1). However, not all CVD RFs are affected to a similar extent and sometimes the clinical benefits can be concealed by the consumption of cardioprotective medications.

a) **Fat mass** In general, ET and incremental PA do not lead to spectacular sustained fat mass losses in obese individuals. For example, a six-month PA or ET intervention in obese individuals results in an average body weight loss of 2 kg [4]. In addition, the maintenance of a reduced body weight during

Table 7.1 Effect of physical activity and exercise training on cardiovascular risk factors, and how to adjust the exercise prescription as a function of the cardiovascular risk

CVD risk factor	Currently observed effects of PA or exercise intervention	How to increase the effects of PA or exercise intervention on the target risk factor
Fat mass	Significant but small reductions	Maximize energy expenditure by sufficiently long, frequent, and intense exercise
Blood pressure	Significant and clinically relevant reductions	Achieve at least moderate-intensity and sufficiently long exercise sessions; add isometric strength training
Blood lipid profile	Significant improvements noticed	Achieve >900 kcal of energy expenditure per week; add sufficiently intense strength training
Glycaemic control	Significant large improvements in glycaemic control in T2DM. Overall positive cardiovascular effects noticed in T1DM	For T2DM: increase the exercise frequency and add high-volume strength training For T1DM: all exercises can be performed, according to general guidelines, but the main focus remains on preventing hypoglycaemia and preserving optimal HbA1c
Inflammation	Significant reductions in blood CRP and IL-6 are observed	To be determined

PA, physical activity; T2DM, type 2 diabetes mellitus; T1DM, type 1 diabetes mellitus; CRP, C-reactive protein; IL-6, interleukin-6.

long-term follow-up is difficult, as body weight regain is very common in this population [5]. However, clinical experience shows that patients adhering to lifestyle intervention are (more) successful in reducing and maintaining a lower body fat mass. Moreover, it is well established that exercise interventions, such as RT, may also lead to incremental increases in lean tissue mass, resulting in either no change in body weight or an apparently unfavourable change [6]. However, on average, after 12 weeks of moderate intensity endurance training or high-intensity interval training (HIIT) whole-body fat mass losses of approximately 1 kg and 1.5 kg respectively are often achieved in obese adults [7]. This corresponds to a reduction of about 1–2% in whole-body fat mass [7]. Therefore, even when the impact of ET on lean tissue mass is taken into account, only small reductions in whole-body fat mass are observed in obese individuals. As a result, ET often leads to disappointingly small reductions in whole-body fat mass in obese individuals. Thus it is to select optimal exercise modalities and to include a dietary intervention to maximize this fat mass loss. Importantly, PA and ET in overweight or obesity improve dietary interventions as follows: (1) greater improvement in BP, glycaemic control, and lipid profile; (2) incremental increase or maintenance of muscle mass and strength; (3) increased endurance and functional capacity; (4) enhanced HRQol. In addition, improvement in endurance capacity, which is only achieved by ET, are related to significant decreases in mortality in obese individuals [8]. In contrast, changes in body mass index are not related to changes in mortality in obese individuals [8], which emphasizes the importance of exercise as a key lifestyle intervention.

b) **Blood pressure** On average ET reduces systolic and diastolic BP by approximately 5 mmHg and 3 mmHg, respectively, in mainly Caucasian cohorts [9]. Even greater reductions in BP are noticed in African and Asian populations (9 mmHg and 5 mmHg for systolic and diastolic BP, respectively) [10]. These effects are clinically relevant and are greater in hypertensive patients who are not (already) taking BP-lowering medications. In fact, PA and exercise intervention is as effective in reducing systolic BP as angiotensin-converting enzyme (ACE) inhibitors, adrenergic receptor blockers, beta-blockers, and/or diuretics [11]. Medication should be started in addition to lifestyle interventions for patients with arterial hypertension (HTN) grade 2 or 3, since lifestyle interventions alone will not generally reduce BP levels to the normal range. A combination of ACE inhibitors or angiotensin II type 1(AT_1) receptor antagonists and calcium-channel blockers should be the first choice for exercising individuals, and a diuretic or spironolactone may be added. Beta-blockers should be restricted to patients with acute myocardial infarction (AMI), HF, or atrial fibrillation (AF), or women wishing to become pregnant. Importantly, while ACE inhibitors/AT_1 receptor antagonists, calcium-channel blockers, and spironolactone are neutral with respect the effects of lifestyle interventions, diuretics and beta-blockers should be avoided because of negative effects on glycaemic control and body weight reduction, respectively.

c) **Blood lipid profile** PA and ET are effective in improving blood lipid profile in healthy people, as shown by increases in high-density lipoprotein cholesterol concentrations (on average by 2 mg/dl) and reductions in blood triglyceride concentrations (on average by 5 mg/dl), although individual effects of up to 50% may be observed [12]. When there is risk of an elevated CVD (e.g. overweight and dyslipidaemia), reductions in blood low-density lipoprotein (on average by 12 mg/dl) may be expected [12]. Exercise maintains its effects even in patients receiving statin medication [13], but the effects of PA and ET are often concealed in these individuals. Nonetheless, their clinical effect of reducing CV events is maintained.

d) **Glycaemic control** PA and ET are highly effective in improving glycaemic control for both type 1 and type 2 diabetes mellitus (DM) patients, as evidenced by significant reductions in blood glycated haemoglobin (HbA1c) concentrations, on average by 0.7% for type 1 and 0.4% for type 2 [14,15]. Hypoglycaemia is a key side effect of exercise, but is primarily observed in type 1 DM, or in type 2 DM when the patient is dependent on insulin medication. Therefore the dose of blood-glucose-lowering medications should be adapted in these patients to avoid hypoglycaemia, which may be observed even up to 12 hours post-exercise. ET acutely reduces glycaemic variability (smaller glucose excursions during the day or coefficient of variability), which is highly advantageous in DM patients [16].

e) **Inflammation** Exercise acutely increases inflammatory markers. However, chronic PA and ET lead to significant reductions in high-sensitivity C-reactive protein (hs-CRP) concentrations in blood, especially when reductions in body mass index or body fat mass are achieved [17]. Blood interleukin-6 concentrations decrease as a result of these lifestyle interventions, but the impact on blood tumour necrosis factor alpha is inconclusive [18].

Overall endurance and resistance exercises have positive effects on CV RFs, with the former having high overall effects. Individual adaptation depends on genetics as well as on individual training adaptations and adherence. As a result, different exercises should be prescribed for each CV RF, and followed individually to monitor short-, mid-, and long-term effects [19]. If the individual response to lifestyle intervention is poor or insufficient to meet RF target ranges, pharmacological treatment must be added.

How to prescribe exercise for improvement of CVD risk factors

Clinicians should start with general exercise recommendations for maintaining or improving CV health. These guidelines state that individuals with an elevated CV risk should perform at least 150 min of aerobic exercise at a moderate intensity (64–76% of peak HR or 12–13 on the 20-point Borg scale), or at least 75 min of high-intensity exercise (77–93% of peak HR or 14–16 on the 20-point Borg scale) on three to five days a week [3]. In addition to these exercises, moderate-intensity strength or RT exercises (60–80% of one-repetition maximum) should be executed on two days a week, targeting the large muscle groups (three series of 8–12 repetitions for each muscle group) [3]. This exercise prescription is adapted further depending on which

CVD RF is positive (see Table 7.1) [19]. It should be noted that these are target exercise prescriptions, which may not be achieved by sedentary, untrained, or obese individuals in the first 1–2 months. Therefore crucial to start with lower-intensity exercise recommendations (e.g. 5–10 min daily to ensure adherence) and subsequently increase duration and intensity on an individual basis, depending on adherence to the exercise prescription.

Exercise prescription and physical activity advice depend on the targets.

a) **Fat mass** The single most important factor predicting fat mass loss as a result of PA or ET is total energy expenditure (EE). Therefore the weekly aerobic exercise volume must be increased significantly (optimally to 250 min, equivalent to an EE >1500 kcal), and clinicians should monitor the EE achieved to verify whether this target is reached. Moderate-intensity (moderate effort) aerobic exercises involving large muscle groups (e.g. walking, stepping, rowing, cross-training) are a logical choice for achieving these these high ET volumes, and an elevated exercise frequency to ensure that exercise sessions are not too long may also be helpful. Obese individuals should be stimulated to increase their habitual PA, in addition to these structured exercise sessions, and aim to maintain an increased PA level. A pedometer could be offered for this purpose. Low-intensity aerobic exercise in obese persons will have less effects on EE and fat mass loss, but should still be introduced to increase adherence and improve overall metabolic adaptations in addition to weight loss. The addition of RT (60–70% of one repetition maximum (RM), and 12–15 repetitions for three series of each exercise targeting large muscle groups) does not facilitate fat mass loss, but does result in favourable changes in muscle mass and strength, basal metabolic rate, and blood lipid profile. It is important to monitor (worsening) orthopaedic symptoms in obese individuals, and adjust the exercise prescription when indicated to prevent dropout due to injuries.

Blood pressure The intensity and session duration of endurance exercise is important to ensure that PA or ET has a significant impact on BP. At least moderate intensity and a target session duration of 30–45 min should be achieved. At the beginning of the programme, exercise can be started with several short sessions daily of, for example, 5 min each. There is some limited evidence indicating that higher exercise intensities (as applied during high-intensity interval training) may be more effective for improving BP, but more data are needed to verify this. Importantly, this training is limited to those individuals with normal exercise responses during exercise. Since the impact of exercise on BP is short-lived (up to 12–24 hours), it is also important to achieve a sufficiently high weekly exercise frequency (daily exercise is preferred). Data also show that the addition of static or isometric RT using handgrip ET at low intensity (40% of one maximal volitional contraction) performed as several intermittent bouts of handgrip contractions lasting 2 min each for a total of 12–15 min per session, could lower BP further. In patients with HTN, it is important to monitor BP responses during exercise to avoid excessive increases in BP (systolic BP >200 mmHg) and maximize the medical safety of ET. For this purpose, ergometry should be performed before starting an exercise programme.

b) **Blood lipid profile** Maximization of the benefits of PA or ET on blood lipid profile requires achievement of a weekly EE of at least 900 kcal. According to a meta-regression analysis, prolongation of the exercise session is particularly beneficial in this regard. In addition, there is some evidence suggesting that the addition of sufficiently intense strength training further facilitates the increase in blood HDL cholesterol. About 5% of patients for whom statins have been prescribed may develop a statin-induced myopathy, which is experienced as muscle soreness or cramps. In such cases, dose and statin should be adapted, and alternatives (e.g. ezetimibe and PCSK9-inhibitors) should be considered.

c) **Glycaemic control** In patients with type 2 DM, it is essential that a high exercise frequency is achieved (at least five days/week), and evidence is accumulating that high-intensity interval training may be more effective in lowering blood HbA1c than moderate-intensity endurance training. However, the medical safety of high-intensity interval training in patients with type 2 DM needs to be established. The addition of strength training exercises facilitates reduction in blood HbA1c; at least 21 sets (three sets for seven muscle groups) should be executed. Exercise programmes for patients with type 1 DM are different as their primary aim is not to improve HbA1c per se, but rather to introduce and increase exercise without provoking hypoglycaemia. Most importantly, it is recommended that, for those patients who experience hypoglycaemia during or after exercise, high-intensity endurance exercises (sprint exercises; e.g. three times 20 seconds) or high-intensity strength exercises (up to 80% of one-repetition maximum) should be added at the end of the training session. This will stabilize the blood glucose concentration following exercise, but may not be sufficient to prevent hypoglycaemia several hours after exercise. Therefore blood glucose monitoring is crucial in these physically active individuals. Modern antidiabetic medication (e.g. DPP-4 inhibitors, GLP1 agonists, and SGLT2 inhibitors) are better tolerated regarding hypoglycaemia and should be preferred in type 2 DM. GLP1 agonists and SGLT2 inhibitors may also have a positive influence on weight reduction. Glinides or sulfonylureas should not be used. Close monitoring of blood glucose concentrations during and after exercise is advocated for patients injecting insulin, and medication prescription should be adjusted according to the planned exercise to avoid hypoglycaemia.

d) **Inflammation** How to chronically lower circulatory markers of inflammation by adapting the training modalities remains to be addressed in future studies. Weight loss is certainly more effective than ET alone. Based on a limited amount of evidence, blood IL-6 concentrations seem to decrease more when the number of training sessions is increased and/or the exercise is prolonged [20].

Tailoring the exercise prescription: a practical approach

Even though RF-specific PA guidelines have been developed, it is evident that different CVD RFs require different exercise prescription strategies to maximize the clinical benefits. Figure 7.1 displays how exercise prescription should be tailored for patients with elevated CVD risk [21].

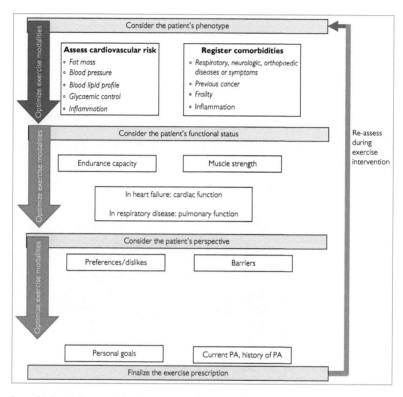

Figure 7.1 Practical approach to tailoring an exercise prescription.

Conclusion

PA and ET are effective in improving the CV risk profile, and hence contribute to the primary prevention of CVD. However, the exercise prescription should be adjusted to target specific CV RFs, and the exercise intervention should be tailored to the individual to optimize clinical benefits and medical safety.

References

1. Lear SA, Hu W, Rangarajan S, et al. The effect of physical activity on mortality and cardiovascular disease in 130 000 people from 17 high-income, middle-income, and low-income countries: the PURE study. *Lancet* 2017; 390: 2643–54.

2. Ekelund U, Tarp J, Steene-Johannessen J, et al. Dose–response associations between accelerometry measured physical activity and sedentary time and all cause mortality: systematic review and harmonised meta-analysis. *BMJ* 2019; 366: l4570.

3. Piepoli MF, Hoes AW, Agewall S, et al. 2016 European Guidelines on cardiovascular disease prevention in clinical practice. The Sixth Joint Task Force of the European Society of Cardiology and Other Societies on Cardiovascular Disease Prevention in Clinical Practice. . *Eur Heart J* 2016; 37: 2315–81.

4. Franz MJ, vanWormer JJ, Crain AL, et al. Weight-loss outcomes: a systematic review and meta-analysis of weight-loss clinical trials with a minimum 1-year follow-up. *J Am Diet Assoc* 2007; 107: 1755–67.

5. Dombrowski SU, Knittle K, Avenell A, et al. Long term maintenance of weight loss with non-surgical interventions in obese adults: systematic review and meta-analyses of randomised controlled trials. *BMJ* 2014; 348: g2646.

6. Batsis JA, Gill LE, Masutani RK, et al. Weight loss interventions in older adults with obesity: a systematic review of randomized controlled trials since 2005. *J Am Geriatr Soc* 2017; 65: 257–68.

7. Keating SE, Johnson NA, Mielke GI, et al. A systematic review and meta-analysis of interval training versus moderate-intensity continuous training on body adiposity. *Obes Rev* 2017; 18(8): 943–64.

8. Lee DC, Sui X, Artero EG, et al. Long-term effects of changes in cardiorespiratory fitness and body mass index on all-cause and cardiovascular disease mortality in men: the Aerobics Center Longitudinal Study. *Circulation* 2011; 124: 2483–90.

9. Williamson W, Foster C, Reid H, et al. Will exercise advice be sufficient for treatment of young adults with prehypertension and hypertension? A systematic review and meta-analysis. *Hypertension* 2016; 68: 78–87.

10. Bersaoui M, Baldew SM, Cornelis N, et al. The effect of exercise training on blood pressure in African and Asian populations: a systematic review and meta-analysis of randomized controlled trials. *Eur J Prev Cardiol* 2019; 26: 1534–44.

11. Naci H, Salcher-Konrad M, Dias S, et al. How does exercise treatment compare with antihypertensive medications? A network meta-analysis of 391 randomised controlled trials assessing exercise and medication effects on systolic blood pressure. *Br J Sports Med* 2019; 53: 859–69.

12. Lin X, Zhang X, Guo J, et al. Effects of exercise training on cardiorespiratory fitness and biomarkers of cardiometabolic health: a systematic review and meta-analysis of randomized controlled trials. *J Am Heart Assoc* 2015; 4: e002014.

13. Gui YJ, Liao CX, Liu Q, et al. Efficacy and safety of statins and exercise combination therapy compared to statin monotherapy in patients with dyslipidaemia: a systematic review and meta-analysis. *Eur J Prev Cardiol* 2017; 24: 907–16.

14. Umpierre D, Ribeiro PA, Kramer CK, et al. Physical activity advice only or structured exercise training and association with HbA1c levels in type 2 diabetes: a systematic review and meta-analysis. *JAMA* 2011; 305: 1790–9.

15. Ostman C1, Jewiss D, King N, et al. Clinical outcomes to exercise training in type 1 diabetes: a systematic review and meta-analysis. *Diabetes Res Clin Pract* 2018; 139: 380–91.

16. Figueira FR, Umpierre D, Casali KR, et al. Aerobic and combined exercise sessions reduce glucose variability in type 2 diabetes: crossover randomized trial. *PLoS One* 2013; 8: e57733.

17. Fedewa MV, Hathaway ED, Ward-Ritacco CL, et al. Effect of exercise training on C reactive protein: a systematic review and meta-analysis of randomised and non-randomised controlled trials. *Br J Sports Med* 2017; 51: 670–6.

18. Monteiro-Junior RS, de Tarso Maciel-Pinheiro P, da Matta Mello Portugal E, et al. Effect of exercise on inflammatory profile of older persons: systematic review and meta-analyses. *J Phys Act Health* 2018; 15: 64–71.

19. Hansen D, Niebauer J, Cornelissen V, et al. Exercise prescription in patients with different combinations of cardiovascular disease risk factors: a consensus statement from the EXPERT Working Group. *Sports Med* 2018; 48: 1781–97.

20. Hayashino Y, Jackson JL, Hirata T, et al. Effects of exercise on C-reactive protein, inflammatory cytokine and adipokine in patients with type 2 diabetes: a meta-analysis of randomized controlled trials. *Metabolism* 2014; 63: 431–40.
21. Hansen D, Piepoli MF, Doehner W. The importance of rehabilitation in the secondary prevention of cardiovascular disease. *Eur J Prev Cardiol* 2019; 26: 273–6.

Further reading

Ambrosetti M, Abreu A, Corrà U, et al. Secondary prevention through comprehensive cardiac re-habilitation: from knowledge to implementation. 2020 update. A position paper from the Secondary Prevention and Rehabilitation Section of the European Association of Preventive Cardiology. *Eur J Prev Cardiol 2020*; e-pub ahead of print.

Chapter 8

Exercise training for low-risk patients

Matthias Wilhelm

Summary

Low-risk cardiac patients should start exercise training (ET) as early as possible after the index event to maintain or improve their cardiorespiratory fitness, muscular strength, and prognosis. Ideally, ET is provided within a multidisciplinary cardiovascular rehabilitation (CR) programme. It can be delivered as an early outpatient or home-based (HB) programme or as a combination of the two approaches, based on patient preference and local facilities. ET should be prescribed on an individual basis after careful clinical and functional assessment, including risk stratification, evaluation of fitness level, behavioural characteristics, personal goals, and exercise preferences. Importantly, the programme should empower the patient for individual long-term physical activity and ET. Aerobic endurance training three to five times weekly should be prescribed, with a goal of at least 150 min of moderate to vigorous exercise per week. Resistance training (RT) twice to three times weekly should also be prescribed. The initial duration and intensity of ET should be adapted to the patient's condition and gradually increased.

59

Introduction

ET is a structured intervention to improve or maintain one or more attributes of physical fitness. It is a core component of multidisciplinary CR programmes and usually comprises aerobic endurance training and dynamic resistance exercise [1]. Flexibility and coordination training are less standardized components which may also be added. Low-risk patients (Box 8.1) include patients after elective percutaneous coronary intervention (PCI), uneventful acute coronary syndrome, and primary PCI, coronary artery bypass grafting, or valve surgery. These patients should start ET as soon as possible after the index event to maintain or improve their cardiorespiratory fitness, muscular strength, and prognosis. ET can be delivered in an early outpatient CR programme or as a HB programme or a combination of the two approaches, based on patient preference and local facilities. mHealth applications and fitness trackers may help to monitor and guide non-supervised ET. Early outpatient

Box 8.1 Characteristics of low-risk patients

- No symptoms of clinical instability (CCS 0, NYHA I, no palpitations or dizziness).
- No severely reduced exercise capacity (>50% of predicted value).
- No LV dysfunction.
- No complex arrhythmias.
- No signs of residual ischaemia (e.g. incomplete revascularization or diffuse disease).
- No uncontrolled arterial hypertension.
- Absence of comorbidities such as CDK, COPD, or DM.
- No ICD or CRT-D/P implantation.

CCS, Canadian Cardiovascular Society grading of angina pectoris; NYHA, New York Heart Association; LV, left ventricular; CKD, chronic kidney disease; COPD, chronic obstructive pulmonary disease; DM, diabetes mellitus; ICD, implantable cardioverter defibrillator; CRT-D/P, cardiac resynchronization therapy with ICD or pacemaker

programmes usually last 8–12 weeks but can be continued in a more flexible model based on patient preferences, fitness level, and health insurance cover [2].

Assessment of low-risk patients

Prior to commencing an ET programme, low-risk status has to be confirmed in a clinical and functional assessment. A careful medical history, clinical examination, and symptom-limited exercise test should be performed.

Symptom-limited exercise test

If the clinical assessment and the review of diagnostic tests (ECG, echocardiography, angiography) suggest a low-risk situation, a cardiopulmonary ET is not mandatory. Standard ergometry can be performed on a cycle ergometer or a treadmill, based on patient preference and available facilities. Optimally, the ET modality should match the aerobic ET modality (Table 8.1). The rate–pressure product (product of maximum heart rate (HR) and systolic blood pressure (BP)) is a surrogate for myocardial oxygen uptake [3] and is used, with others, as an indicator for a maximum test:

- rate–pressure product >20 000–25 000 bpm × mmHg
- rate of perceived exertion ≥18 (based on the Borg Scale 6–20)
- patient appearing exhausted.

The aims of the exercise test are to:

- determine maximum exercise capacity
- detect signs of exercise-induced myocardial ischaemia or arrhythmias
- evaluate the haemodynamic response to an exercise stimulus (BP, HR profile) under pharmacological therapy
- determine the optimal training intensity zones for endurance exercise.

Table 8.1 Choosing an exercise testing protocol for low-risk patients		
	Bicycle ergometer	Treadmill
Test duration goal	8–12 min	8–12 min
Haemodynamic monitoring	BP, HR, rate–pressure product, 12 lead ECG	
Protocol	Ramp protocols Starting at 20–50 watts and increasing by 10–20 watts/min	Bruce or modified Bruce protocol Starting at 3.2 km/h, 10% or 3.2 km/h 0% grade 3 min stages, increasing by 1.6 km/h and 2% grade
Indication	Patient preference Gait problems, Planned exercise training on a bicycle ergometer	Patient preference Obese patients with sitting problems Planned exercise training on a treadmill Rate-adaptive pacemaker

Source data from Fletcher GF, Ades PA, Kligfield P, et al. Exercise standards for testing and training: A scientific statement from the American heart association. *Circulation* 2013; 128: 873-934.

Definition of exercise training goals

Exercise test results are crucial for the definition of individualized ET intensity zones and goals for the ET programme. General objectives are to:

- improve a reduced exercise capacity or stabilize a normal exercise capacity
- monitor the response of the cardiovascular (CV) system to a prolonged exercise stimulus (HR, BP, arrhythmias)
- educate the patient on how to approximate the relative intensity during any given exercise
- empower the patient to perform non-supervised exercise and to adhere to ET recommendations in the long term
- contribute to weight-loss interventions in obese patients.

Prescription for aerobic endurance training

Outpatient CR programmes usually offer two or three supervised ET sessions per week. Based on the patient's condition and preferences, and the equipment available in the CR facility, several modes of aerobic endurance training are applicable (Table 8.2). Patients may gradually increase their ET frequency to five or more session per week, including non-supervised ET sessions. Initial training intensity and duration should be individualized based on patient characteristics. ET can be prescribed based on the FITT principle [4]:

- frequency—number of ET sessions per week
- intensity—percentage peak workload (%peak watts), percentage heart rate reserve (%HRR), and/or rate of perceived exertion (RPE) (HHR is not recommended in

Table 8.2 Common aerobic endurance training modes

Mode	Characteristics	Monitoring
Walking	Suitable for obese or previously untrained patients with low cardiorespiratory fitness No special equipment required. Walking speed determines ET intensity (brisk walking corresponds to moderate-intensity exercise)	HR, RPE
Nordic walking	Using poles includes additional muscle groups of the arms Poles may increase safety in elderly patients with gait problems Poles allow faster walking at higher exercise intensity	HR, RPE
Jogging	Most effective form of aerobic endurance exercise Can be simulated with treadmill training that is more suitable for group training of patients with different fitness levels Restricted to patients with higher fitness levels Should be started gradually in novices and obese patients due to strain on lower-extremity joints and tendons	HR, RPE
Bicycle exercise training	Stationary devices are suitable for group training and allow monitoring of BP and HR, including ECG recording (not mandatory in stable low-risk patients) Exercise intensity is easily adjustable based on watts Outdoor cycling may be an enjoyable option for selected patients at a later stage of non-supervised exercise Electric bicycles allow outdoor cycling for patients with lower levels of fitness Risk of traffic accidents	watts, HR, RPE

Reproduced from Vanhees L, Rauch B, Piepoli M, et al. Importance of characteristics and modalities of physical activity and exercise in the management of cardiovascular health in individuals with cardiovascular disease (part iii). *Eur J Prev Cardiol* 2012;19:1333-1356 with permission from SAGE Publishing.

cardiac patients because a meaningful peak HR is difficult to obtain (e.g. beta-blocker therapy, non-maximal exercise test after a cardiac event)) (Table 8.3)
- time—duration of ET session
- type—exercises that involve large muscle groups (e.g. walking, running, bicycle riding).

Table 8.3 Characteristics of endurance exercise intensity domains				
Endurance exercise intensity domain	Very light to light	Light to moderate	Moderate to high	High to severe
Training protocol	Continuous	Continuous	Continuous	Interval
Relation to lactate or ventilatory thresholds	Below the first threshold	Near or slightly above the first threshold	Between thresholds or near the second threshold	Above the second threshold
%HRR or peak watts	≤40	40–60	60–80	≥80
RPE (20 point scale)	≤10	11–12	13–14	≥15

HRR is calculated from the difference between peak and resting HR. HR-derived training zones are calculated by adding a certain percentage of the HRR to the resting HR (see Figure 8.1 for an example).

Source data from Mezzani A, Hamm LF, Jones AM, et al. Aerobic exercise intensity assessment and prescription in cardiac rehabilitation: A joint position statement of the European Association for Cardiovascular Prevention and Rehabilitation, The American Association of Cardiovascular and Pulmonary Rehabilitation and The Canadian Association of Cardiac Rehabilitation. *Eur J Prev Cardiol* 2013;20:442-467.

Binder RK, Wonisch M, Corra U, et al. Methodological approach to the first and second lactate threshold in incremental cardiopulmonary exercise testing. *Eur J Cardiovasc Prev Rehabil* 2008;15:726-734.

Sedentary or very deconditioned patients should start with 5–10 min of very light to light-intensity aerobic exercise. Fitter patients (>80% of predicted values) will tolerate 20 min of light- to moderate-intensity aerobic exercise. Determination of training intensity depends on the training modality (e.g. %HRR for walking, Nordic walking and running, %peak watts for cycle ergometer training). Given documented improvement (e.g. toleration of the same training load with a lower HR and/or RPE), exercise intensity can be up-titrated (Figure 8.1). The goal for maintenance is 30–60 min of moderate- to high-intensity aerobic exercise per session [5,6] (see Table 8.6 in the section on prescription for dynamic resistance training).

RPE based on the Borg Scale is a useful alternative to HR or workload for long-term surveillance of training intensity, especially for patients who are reluctant to wear HR monitors. Limitations, such as psychological factors, increased ambition, and group dynamics, have to be respected. The appropriateness of RPE can be supported with simple rules like 'hear your breathing but be able to talk' as an indicator for moderate-intensity exercise [6].

Aerobic endurance training protocols

Moderate-intensity continuous exercise (MICE), range from low to moderate to moderate to high intensity) is the standard ET protocol in low-risk cardiac patients. Protocols usually start with a 5 min warm-up phase with an intensity below the first threshold, followed by the ET phase of 20–50 min between the first and second threshold, and finish with a 5 min cool-down phase (Figure 8.1, A and B) [5,6].

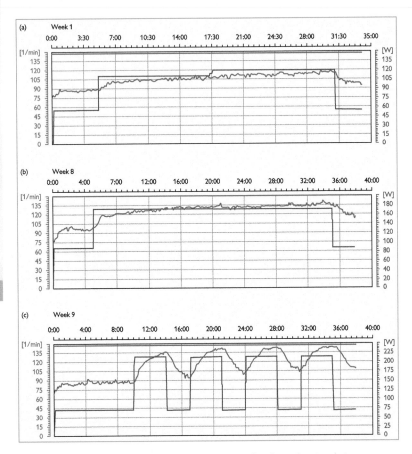

Figure 8.1 Representative aerobic endurance training sessions for a low-risk patient during a 12-week cardiac rehabilitation programme: red, heart rate; blue, training load (watts). The patient was a 58-year-old man with a non-ST-elevation myocardial infarction and left ventricular ejection fraction 62%. A bicycle ergometry was performed. The maximum exercise capacity was 222 watts (95% of predicted), resting heart rate 60 bpm, peak HR 162 bpm (99% of predicted), rate–pressure product 32 400 bpm×mmHg, and RPE 19–20 on the Borg Scale. Definition of MICE training zone: (a) 50–80% peak watts, 110–176 watts; (b) 50–80% HRR, 110–140 bpm, RPE 11–14 on the 6–20 Borg Scale.

(a) First MICE training, starting at 110 watts. Exercise intensity level was checked at the middle of the session. Since the patient reported an RPE of 10, the workload was increased to 120 watts. Peak HR reached 122 bpm and the RPE was 12.

(b) Over 8 weeks of MICE training, the workload could be increased to 170 watts. Peak HR reached 137 bpm and the RPE was 14.

(c) In week 9, HIIT was introduced at the patient's request. For the last three weeks of the programme, two HIIT sessions and one MICE session per week were performed. A workload above and below the MICE zone was chosen for the high- and low-intensity intervals (220 watts and 75 watts). The appropriateness of the protocol was controlled with HR and RPE at the end of the first low-intensity interval (goal, below MICE zone: HR 95 bpm and RPE 10), and at the end of the fourth high-intensity interval (goal, above MICE zone: HR 144 bpm and RPE 16).

High-intensity interval training (HIIT), also called aerobic interval training, is an effective alternative to MICE for selected low-risk patients. A commonly used protocol starts with a 10 minute warm-up phase with an intensity below the first threshold, followed by four 4 minute high-intensity intervals above the second threshold, interrupted by 3 minute recovery intervals below the first threshold (Figure 8.1c). No superior benefits with regard to improvement of exercise capacity compared with properly adjusted MICE training are to be expected. Some patients appreciate the experience of high-intensity intervals for regaining confidence and the fact that the protocol is more diverse than MICE [5,6]. However, others may not like the feeling of near exhaustion over several minutes and several intervals.

Prescription for dynamic resistance training

Aerobic endurance training should be complemented by two or three sessions of dynamic RT during the outpatient CR programme [6,7]. Like endurance training, it can be prescribed based on the FITT principle [4]. Dynamic RT is less suitable for group training in the initial phase, where exercises should be individually supervised as the correct technique is essential. Single and/or dual limb movements should be adjusted according to the patient's individual skill level [6]. The resistance exercise equipment may vary considerably in cost, complexity of operational skill/coordination, and time efficiency. Free weights and weight machine training have distinct characteristics (Table 8.4). The key is to select the appropriate equipment for supervised and unsupervised training that is safe, effective, and accessible [7].

Table 8.4 Dynamic resistance training modes

Mode	Characteristics	Monitoring
Free weights	Resistance is applied using a freely moving body (e.g. barbells, dumbbells, medicine balls, bodyweight) ET challenges the patient to control, stabilize and direct the movement	RPE, % of 1 RM possible for barbells and dumbbells
Weight machines	Resistance is applied in a guided or restricted manner (e.g. plate-loaded devices, rubber-bands) ET aids the patient to keep balance and equilibrium and can easily be adjusted to varying resistances Reduces the likelihood of injury	% of 1 RM, RPE

1 RM, one repetition maximum; RPE, rate of perceived exertion.

Source data from Vanhees L, Rauch B, Piepoli M, et al. Importance of characteristics and modalities of physical activity and exercise in the management of cardiovascular health in individuals with cardiovascular disease (part iii). *Eur J Prev Cardiol* 2012;19:1333-1356.

Williams MA, Haskell WL, Ades PA, et al. Resistance exercise in individuals with and without cardiovascular disease: 2007 update: A scientific statement from the American Heart Association Council on Clinical Cardiology and Council on Nutrition, physical activity, and metabolism. *Circulation* 2007;116:572-584.

The general recommendations for RT are as follows [7]:

- it should be performed in a rhythmical manner at a moderate to slow controlled speed through a full range of motion
- breath-holding and straining (Valsalva manoeuvre) should be avoided by exhaling during the exertion phase and inhaling during the relaxation phase
- training of upper- and lower-body muscle groups should be alternated to allow adequate rest between exercises
- the major muscle groups of the upper and lower extremities should be involved (e.g. chest press, shoulder press, triceps extension, biceps curl, pull-down (upper back), lower-back extension, abdominal crunch/curl-up, quadriceps extension or leg press, leg curls (hamstrings), and calf raise)
- it should be limited to a single set performed on 2-3 non consecutive days per week.

The appropriate limb-specific training weight loads are obtained by determining the maximum weight that can be lifted during a given exercise (1-RM). An initial intensity that corresponds to 30–40% of 1-RM for the upper body and 50–60% of 1-RM for the hips and legs is recommended. As the individual progresses, the exercise load can be increased to 50–80% of 1-RM to further improve muscular strength and endurance. When the determination of 1-RM is deemed inappropriate, the load–repetition relationship for RT can be approximated (Table 8.5). The goal for strength maintenance is one set of 10–15 repetitions (60–80% 1-RM) for 8–10 dynamic resistance exercises on two to three days per week [6,7] (Table 8.6).

Table 8.5 Characteristics of dynamic resistance training domains			
Resistance exercise intensity domain	Low	Moderate	High
Training objective	Enhance muscular endurance	Enhance power and strength	Enhance power and strength
Maximum possible repetitions	>15	8–15	<8
%1-RM	<60%	60–80%	>80%
RPE (20-point scale)	≤10	11–14	≥15

1-RM, one repetition maximum; RPE, rate of perceived exertion.

Source data from Vanhees L, Rauch B, Piepoli M, et al. Importance of characteristics and modalities of physical activity and exercise in the management of cardiovascular health in individuals with cardiovascular disease (part iii). *Eur J Prev Cardiol* 2012;19:1333-1356.

Williams MA, Haskell WL, Ades PA, et al. Resistance exercise in individuals with and without cardiovascular disease: 2007 update: A scientific statement from the American Heart Association Council on Clinical Cardiology and Council on Nutrition, physical activity, and metabolism. *Circulation* 2007;116:572-584.

Table 8.6 Summary of aerobic endurance and dynamic resistance training in low-risk cardiac patients

	Stage	Frequency	Intensity*	Time	Type
Aerobic endurance training	Initial	3 days/week	Light-to-moderate (MICE)	10–20 min	Walking, Nordic walking, jogging, bicycle riding
	Maintenance	5 days/week	Moderate-to-high (MICE) or intermittent high (HIIT)	30-60 min	
Dynamic resistance training	Initial	2 days/week	Low	One set of 8–10 exercises	Training on weight machines or with free weights including large muscle groups of the trunk and the upper and lower extremities
	Maintenance	2–3 days/ week (not consecutive)	Moderate	One set of 8–10 exercises	

*See Tables 8.3 and 8.5.

Precautions and safety in exercise training for low-risk patients

Both research findings and clinical experience indicate that ET is relatively safe in the cohort of cardiac patients with a confirmed low-risk status (Box 8.1) [6]. After a percutaneous intervention, ET can start immediately after the punctured vessel has healed. After cardiac surgery, the programme can start within the first 6 weeks after median thoracotomy. Wound healing and conditions that may alter the low-risk status (e.g. post-operative infection, Dressler syndrome, arrhythmias) should be carefully monitored. Thoracic shear stress and pressure stress must be avoided in the first 6–8 weeks after thoracotomy. There is no scientific evidence available specifying the duration and level of supervision and monitoring for ET in low-risk patients [6]. Whether to allow unsupervised ET should be an individualized and multidisciplinary decision, including the patient's perspective.

Endurance training

There are no specific CV concerns about endurance training after an uneventful maximum exercise test with a normal haemodynamic response. If the endurance training mode is brisk walking, Nordic walking, or jogging, local muscle strain can be avoided by an appropriate warm-up and gradual increasing duration and intensity of training.

Resistance training

Two particular concerns with RT are avoidance of injury (e.g. local muscle strain) and potentially uncontrolled elevation of BP. Factors associated with both injury risk and increased BP are:

- magnitude of the isometric component
- number of repetitions
- load intensity and duration
- amount of muscle mass involved.

These factors must be taken into account in the initial prescription and during the progression of RT, and BP and RPE should be closely monitored. RT should start only after an appropriate warm-up [7].

Conclusion

ET is a corner stone in the holistic management of low risk cardiac patients and should be initiated immediately after the index event. Given the stable cardiac conditions in these patients, early outpatient or home-based ET or a combination thereof are feasible. ET should best be integrated in a multidisciplinary CR programme and be tailored based on patient's preferences, abilities and local facilities. Important components are aerobic endurance training and dynamic RT that should be prescribed according to the FITT principle. During the programme, the patients should be empowered to continue ET in the long-term. mHealth applications and fitness trackers may facilitate the transition from supervised to non-supervised ET and may assist selected patients to adhere to ET recommendations.

References

1. Corrà U, Piepoli MF, Carre F, et al. Secondary prevention through cardiac rehabilitation: physical activity counselling and exercise training. *Eur Heart J* 2010; 31: 1967–74.

2. Piepoli MF, Corrà U, Adamopoulos S, et al. Secondary prevention in the clinical management of patients with cardiovascular diseases. Core components, standards and outcome measures for referral and delivery. *Eur J Prev Cardiol* 2014; 21: 664–81.

3. Fletcher GF, Ades PA, Kligfield P, et al. Exercise standards for testing and training: a scientific statement from the American Heart Association. *Circulation* 2013; 128: 873–934.

4. Garber CE, Blissmer B, Deschenes MR, et al. American College of Sports Medicine position stand. Quantity and quality of exercise for developing and maintaining cardiorespiratory, musculoskeletal, and neuromotor fitness in apparently healthy adults: guidance for prescribing exercise. *Med Sci Sports Exerc* 2011; 43: 1334–59.

5. Mezzani A, Hamm LF, Jones AM, et al. Aerobic exercise intensity assessment and prescription in cardiac rehabilitation. *Eur J Prev Cardiol* 2013; 20: 442–67.

6. Vanhees L, Rauch B, Piepoli M, et al. Importance of characteristics and modalities of physical activity and exercise in the management of cardiovascular health in individuals with cardiovascular disease (part iii). *Eur J Prev Cardiol* 2012; 19: 1333–56.

7. Williams MA, Haskell WL, Ades PA, et al. Resistance exercise in individuals with and without cardiovascular disease: 2007 update. A scientific statement from the American Heart Association Council on Clinical Cardiology and Council on Nutrition, Physical Activity, and Metabolism. *Circulation* 2007; 116: 572–84.

Chapter 9

Exercise training programmes for high-risk and specific groups of patients

Jean-Paul Schmid and Ugo Corrà

Summary

Exercise training (ET) in cardiac patients is considered safe, even early after an acute event or in the case of advanced heart disease. However, clinical incidents during rehabilitation may occur, in particular in patients considered to be 'high risk'. Therefore these patients have to be identified at the beginning of an exercise-based cardiac rehabilitation (CR) programme and deserve particular attention. This includes a thorough clinical assessment, a tailored exercise prescription, and appropriate monitoring.

Introduction

ET improves physical capacity, health-related quality of life (HRQoL), and potentially mortality and hospitalization rate in cardiac patients. This also applies to 'high-risk' patients, i.e. patients after an acute coronary syndrome (ACS) with extended left-ventricular myocardial damage or heart failure (HF) with reduced ejection fraction [1]. ET counteracts negative remodelling after an acute myocardial injury and has the potential to improve left-ventricular function in patients with mild to moderate HF. Even in patients with most advanced left-ventricular dysfunction, such as those treated with a left-ventricular assist device (LVAD), endurance exercise is feasible and safe and helps patients to remain physically active and to participate in an active life.

However, compared with low-risk patients, particular attention in the handling of these patients is required.

Definition of 'high-risk' patients

In the setting of CR, 'high risk' refers to (1) risk of the occurrence of potentially fatal ventricular arrhythmias and (2) risk of left ventricular decompensation or worsening myocardial function.

> **Box 9.1 Markers of 'high-risk' patients**
>
> - Symptoms of advanced disease: dyspnoea, NYHA functional class II–III, or hypotension.
> - Arrhythmias (e.g. atrial fibrillation, non-sustained ventricular tachycardias).
> - Signs of pleural or pericardial effusions.
> - Frailty.
> - Poor exercise capacity (<50% of predicted value).
> - Clinically manifest comorbidities.

Although ET, irrespective of whether it is endurance training or resistance training (RT), has been shown to be safe even in patients with advanced heart disease, the underlying condition can produce a serious complication at any time. We know that the risk of ventricular arrhythmias depends not only on left ventricular function, but also on the structural characteristics of the myocardium (aneurysms, scars, valvular disease, or revascularization status). The clinical condition, i.e. volume status, oxygen saturation, or electrolyte status, must also be taken into account (Box 9.1).

Therefore ET should only be performed in a clinically stable situation after optimization of medical therapy. The shorter the time since clinical stabilization or the more advanced the disease, the higher is the need for supervision and clinical control.

Assessment of high-risk patients

A patient starting endurance exercise requires both clinical stability and minimal exercise capacity (i.e. ability to perform an exercise session for at least 10 min). Early mobilization (EM) during recovery from a major clinical event is the first step towards achieving the necessary functional efficacy and self-confidence to be able to perform a reliable symptom-limited exercise test and start an ET programme.

Clinical assessment

A particularly detailed clinical assessment and summary of the disease history is required for all 'high-risk' patients starting an exercise-based CR programme. In addition to the assessment of the core components common to all clinical conditions [2], the following are particularly important.

Medical history:

a) screening for comorbidities and disabilities (particularly renal function, diabetes mellitus, and musculoskeletal disease)

b) complications of recent surgical interventions, cognitive/neurological impairments, healing wounds, extensive haematoma.

Markers of disease severity:

a) NYHA functional class >II

b) pulmonary congestion, peripheral oedema, hypotension

c) signs of pleural or pericardial effusion

d) distinct dyspnoea and reduced oxygen saturation

e) signs of cachexia and disturbance of balance

f) reduced glomerular filtration rate, disturbance of serum electrolytes, elevated brain natriuretic peptide (BNP).

Functional assessment

After clinical stabilization, before starting a regular ET programme, an appropriate functional assessment is necessary, both at rest and during exercise. This includes a symptom-limited exercise test and, if not recently performed, echocardiography.

Cardiopulmonary exercise testing (CPET) with respiratory gas analysis yields detailed information on cardiopulmonary interaction and adaptation to exercise and provides important prognostic information. It is recommended for all patients with advanced HF and for those in which the exercise prescription will be based on knowledge of the first and second lactate thresholds.

The most frequently used items for prognostic assessment (Figure 9.1) are parameters linked to the functional capacity (e.g. peak VO_2 or early occurrence of the first lactate threshold) (panels 3 and 5). Another very important and sensitive marker is a reduced ventilatory efficiency reflected by an increased VE/VCO_2 slope (panel 4). It indicates a ventilation–perfusion mismatch of either pre- or post-capillary origin or impaired diffusion and correlates, amongst others, with pulmonary congestion. The chronotropic response and stroke volume (the latter determined by means of the oxygen pulse VO_2/HR) are depicted in panel 2. A reduced absolute value or a decrease in the oxygen pulse are signs of left-ventricular suffering during exercise. The inefficient rise of cardiac output produces an oscillatory ventilation pattern (panel 1), a marker of advanced haemodynamic impairment and sensitivity to volume overload. Finally, pulmonary comorbidities are reflected by a reduced tidal volume and high breathing rate (panel 7) as well as exhaustion of the breathing reserve (difference between maximal minute ventilation tested at rest and maximal ventilation during exercise ≤20 L).

The clinical significance of a combination of prognostic parameters derived from CPET has been summarized in a common statement by the European Association of Preventive Cardiology (EAPC) and the American Heart Association (AHA) (Figure 9.2) [3]. The variables in green correspond to normal absolute values or normal behaviour of parameters during CPET and are related to an excellent prognosis (event-free survival in the next 1–4 years >90%). Exercise variables in yellow, orange, or red correspond to a progressive severity of HF and hence a worse prognosis (>50% major adverse events in 1–4 years for variables in red). These patients need particular attention during an ET programme.

Determination of exercise intensity

After an acute cardiac event or surgery, gradual mobilization/calisthenics, respiratory training, and small muscle strength exercise can be considered alone or in

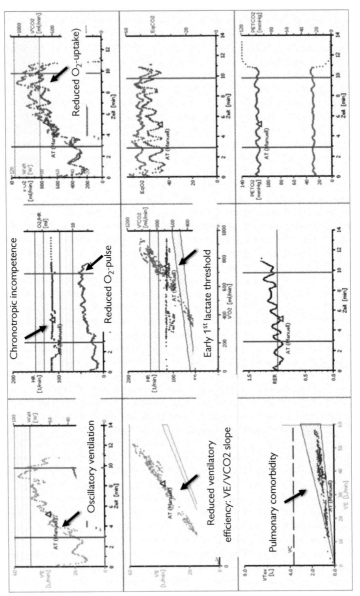

Figure 9.1 Cardiopulmonary exercise stress test for a patient with advanced heart disease: demonstration of different signs of poor prognosis.

Standard ET variables

VE/Vco$_2$ slope	Peak Vo$_2$[a]	EOV	P$_{ET}$-CO$_2$
Ventilatory class I VE/Vco$_2$ slope <30.0	Weber class A Peak Vo$_2$ >20.0 mL O$_2$·kg^{-1}·min^{-1}	Not present	Resting P$_{ET}$-CO$_2$ ≥33.0 mmHg 3–8 mmHg increase during ET
Ventilatory class II VE/Vco$_2$ slope 30.0–35.9	Weber class B Peak Vo$_2$ = 16.0–20.0 mL O$_2$·kg^{-1}·min^{-1}		
Ventilatory class III VE/Vco$_2$ slope 36.0–44.9	Weber class C Peak Vo$_2$ = 10.0–15.9 mL O$_2$·kg^{-1}·min^{-1}	Present	Resting P$_{ET}$-CO$_2$ <33.0 mmHg <3 mmHg increase during exercise
Ventilatory class IV VE/Vco$_2$ slope ≥45.0	Weber class D Peak Vo$_2$ = 100 mL O$_2$·kg^{-1}·min^{-1}		

Haemodynamics	ECG	HRR
Rise in systolic BP during ET	No sustained arrhythmias, ectopic foci, and/or ST segment changes during ET and/or in recovery	>12 beats at 1 min recovery
Flat systolic BP response during exercise	Altered rhythm, ectopic foci, and or ST segment changes during ET and/or in recover: did not lead to test termination	≤12 beats at 1 min recovery
Drop in systolic BP during ET	Altered rhythm, ectopic foci, and/or ST segment changes during ET and/or in recovery: led to test termination	

Patient reason for test termination

Lower extremity muscle fatigue	Angina
	Dyspnoea

Figure 9.2 Prognostic and diagnostic stratification for patients with heart failure based on cardiopulmonary exercise testing data [3]. VE/Vco$_2$, ventilatory efficiency; Vo$_2$, oxygen uptake; EOV, exertional oscillatory ventilation; P$_{ET}$co$_2$, end-tidal carbon dioxide; BP, blood pressure; ET, exercise test; HRR, heart rate reserve.

Reproduced from Guazzi M, Adams V, Conraads V, et al. EACPR and AHA: EACPR/AHA Joint Scientific Statement. Clinical recommendations for cardiopulmonary exercise testing data assessment in specific patient populations. *Eur Heart J* 2012; 33: 2917–27 with permission from Oxford University Press

combination. Each exercise modality should be tested in the individual patient to verify clinical and haemodynamic tolerance, ascertain acceptability, and prove safety. Accordingly, this phase should be extremely flexible in terms of temporal and modality development.

Typically, in this stage of mobilization and clinical stabilization, the training programme is offered in an in-patient setting because of the necessity for:

a) supervision during training sessions and regular evaluation of training response

b) optimization of HR control, particularly in patients with atrial fibrillation (AF) or HF

c) management of clinical symptoms of hypotension, fluid overload, or Dressler syndrome

d) adaptation of drug treatment (diuretics and medication to lower peripheral resistance)

e) identification of signs and symptoms of cardiac decompensation or complications in relation to recent interventional procedures or surgery (for patients with conditions after heart valve surgery and coronary artery bypass grafting or implantation of LVADs or other devices).

In the early stage of mobilization, accomplishment of a symptom-limited exercise test is often not possible or of poor clinical value. Minimal exercise capacity is necessary in order to have some idea about the haemodynamic response to a stress test. There are no strict rules defining a minimal duration, but 3–5 min with a 10 watt ramp protocol on an ergometer should be suitable. The better the exercise capacity, the more reliable the data from the stress test.

Ideally, a CPET is performed to allow a detailed exercise prescription. In addition to providing maximal workload and HR, it enables the first and second lactate thresholds to be determined [4]. This serves as the best basis for exercise prescription (Figure 9.3).

Exercise intensity can be divided into three phases. Phase I corresponds to the recovery zone, which does not show a significant rise in blood lactate with exercise. Phase II corresponds to the zone of light to moderate endurance exercise intensity with a mixed aerobic and anaerobic energy supply and moderate accumulation of lactic acid. Phase III corresponds to the high-intensity exercise zone above the anaerobic threshold and related to a steep increase of blood lactate.

When CPET is not available or the determination of lactate thresholds is not reliable, alternative methods can be used. The subjective rating of perceived exertion (Borg Scale) is the easiest way to guide exercise intensity. However, the method must be carefully introduced to the patients and some training is necessary before it can be applied reliably. Methods based on HR can be influenced by chronotropic incompetence or HR-lowering medication, so they may be less credible. If the HR increase is diminished (HR reserve is low), calculation of the training HR should be based on the 'HR reserve' method (Karvonen formula).

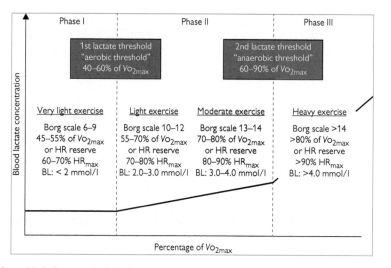

Figure 9.3 Different methods for determining exercise intensity: BL, blood lactate.

Reproduced from Binder RK, Wonisch M, Corra U, et al. Methodological approach to the first and second lactate threshold in incremental cardiopulmonary exercise testing. *Eur J Cardiovasc Prev Rehabil* 2008; 15: 726–34 with permission from SAGE Publishing.

Exercise modalities

In general, the patient's age, concomitant disease(s), leisure and working habits, preferences and abilities, logistical restraints, and the availability of ET facilities and equipment should be taken into account when selecting the exercise modality.

Endurance exercise

Three types of endurance ET have been studied in patients with advanced heart disease (Figure 9.4). Currently, the type used most frequently is the constant workload exercise, typically performed at moderate to high exercise intensities in steady state conditions of aerobic energetic yield, which allows the patient to perform prolonged training sessions (up to 45–60 min duration). It should be started at a low level (50% of peak VO_2) in patients who are unfamiliar with regular exercise or who have a low exercise capacity.

Low-intensity interval training programmes are generally performed on an electrically braked cycle ergometer, which maximizes control over the patient's workload. It provides small stimuli to the skeletal muscle with a very small haemodynamic load and therefore is well tolerated. The primary aim should be to increase the duration from 15 to 30 min, with two or three training sessions per week. Exercise is guided by the perceived intensity of exertion based on maximal exercise parameters or, if available, the first and

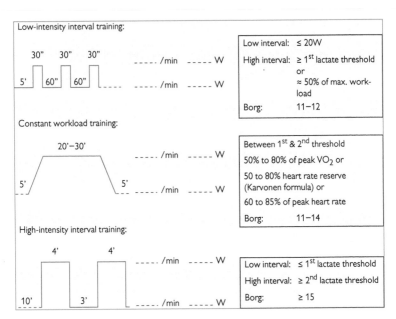

Figure 9.4 Types of endurance exercise training for cardiac patients. Such kind of printed form can be used for training prescription, indicating heart rate and workload of the corresponding exercise intensity.

second lactate threshold. The hard and recovery segments have a duration of 30s and 60s, respectively, and the hard segments are performed at 50% of power output achieved during an incremental bicycle test. Typically, the intensity of the first three hard segments is reduced to allow warm-up. As the patient's exercise capacity improves, the intensity of the hard segments should be increased accordingly. Depending on the work–recovery interval chosen, 10–12 work phases can be performed. After the training intensity has been increased steadily, generally over 4 weeks, patients performing well with low-intensity training can be switched to the steady state workload modality.

Those who tolerate steady state workload training well and can improve their exercise capacity further can be switched to HIIT. It has also been shown to be well tolerated in patients with reduced ejection fraction (EF) and a functional status NYHA class II–III. HIIT generally leads to a greater increase of exercise capacity, at least in the short term, and has the potential to reduce left ventricular dimensions and EF [5–7].

Resistance/strength training

Soon after the positive effects and safety of aerobic endurance exercise in cardiac patients had been ascertained, increasing attention was paid to other training modalities, in particular those aimed at improving reduced muscle strength. These included RT of the peripheral muscles and, more recently, inspiratory muscle training [8].

RT involves muscle contractions against a specific opposing force, such as lifting weights. Earlier concerns about a detrimental effect on left-ventricular function and

Table 9.1 Load repetition relationship for resistance training	
% 1-RM	Repetitions possible
60	17
70	12
80	8
90	5
100	1

Reproduced from Williams MA, Haskell WL, Ades PA, et al. Resistance exercise in individuals with and without cardiovascular disease: 2007 update: a scientific statement from the American Heart Association Council on Clinical Cardiology and Council on Nutrition, Physical Activity, and Metabolism. *Circulation* 2007;116:572-84 with permission from Wolters Kluwer.

negative remodelling have not been confirmed [9]. Since functional alterations in the skeletal muscle are considered an important determinant of exercise intolerance in HF, resistance/strength training should be considered in these patients. However, endurance exercise is the mainstay in HF patients because of the superiority of endurance training on exercise capacity and left ventricular function.

The haemodynamic stress of RT depends on the amount of weight lifted (percentage of 1-RM), the size of the working muscle mass, and the relation between the duration of muscle contraction and the rest period between repetitions.

A maximal strength test (i.e. 1-RM) is generally unsuitable for determining the training intensity for HF patients. Instead, a graded stress test can be applied: the training intensity is set at the level of resistance which the patient can perform for a specified number of times (estimated percentage of 1-RM) (Table 9.1). The load can then be increased progressively according to the Borg Scale. In patients with moderate risk, Borg Scale should be at a maximum rate of perceived exertion of 15–16.

In patients with advanced HF or very low exercise tolerance, RT can safely be applied if small muscle groups are trained, short bouts of work are applied, and the number of repetitions is limited with a work/recovery duration ratio of at least 1:2. Elastic bands (Thera-Band) can also be used suitably, although the effect is difficult to quantify.

RT should be individually adapted to the patient by an experienced exercise therapist under medical supervision, and each patient must be individually introduced to the training regimen (Table 9.2).

a) Step I 'Instruction phase': improves intermuscular coordination and physical perception and gets the patient accustomed to the modality of the exercise. These preparatory exercises are conducted slowly, with very low resistance (<30% 1-RM) until the patient is confident with the course of the movements.

b) Step II 'Resistance/endurance phase': training is started with a high number of repetitions (12–25) at a low intensity (30–40% 1-RM), corresponding to combined endurance/resistance with a low haemodynamic load. When the patient is confident with the exercise, they can proceed to the next phase (strength phase).

c) Step III 'Muscle build-up phase': weights are increased progressively up to 40–60% of 1-RM.

Table 9.2 Recommendations for the implementation of resistance/ strength training in CHF patients

Training programme	Training objective	Intensity	Repetitions	Training volume
Step I: Pretraining	To learn and practice the correct implementation, to learn perception, and to improve intermuscular coordination	<30% 1-RM RPE 12	5–10	2–3 training sessions per week 1–3 circuits during each session
Step II: Resistance/ endurance training	To improve local aerobic endurance and intermuscular coordination	30–40% 1-RM RPE 12–13	12–25	2–3 sessions per week, 1 circuit per session
Step III: Strength training/build up muscles	To increase muscle mass (hypertrophy) and to improve intramuscular coordination	40–60% 1-RM RPE 15	8–15	2–3 sessions per week, 1 circuit per session

Reproduced from Vanhees L, Rauch B, Piepoli M, et al. Importance of characteristics and modalities of physical activity and exercise in the management of cardiovascular health in individuals with cardiovascular disease (part iii). *Eur J Prev Cardiol* 2012;19:1333-1356 with permission from SAGE Publishing.

Inspiratory muscle training

Trials using inspiratory muscle training in HF patients suggest that this intervention can improve exercise capacity and HRQoL, particularly in those who present with inspiratory muscle weakness [11]. Hence, routine screening for inspiratory muscle weakness is advisable, and specific inspiratory muscle training in addition to standard endurance training might be beneficial. It has been suggested that respiratory training should start at 30% of the maximal inspiratory mouth pressure (PI_{max}) and the intensity should be adjusted every 7–10 days up to a maximum of 60% [12]. Training duration should be 20–30 min/day with a frequency of 3–5 sessions per week for a minimum of 8 weeks.

Most studies of congestive heart failure (CHF) have used the Threshold Inspiratory Muscle Trainer (Respironics Health Scan Inc., Cedar Grove, NJ, USA), but devices with the potential to reach higher inspiratory pressures, such as the Power-Breathe (HaB International Ltd, Southam, Warwickshire, UK), might be used when inspiratory muscle strength is preserved.

Specific populations (patients with ICD, CRT, and assist devices)

The literature on exercise in patients with an implantable cardioverter–defibrillator (ICD), receiving cardiac resynchronization therapy (CRT), or with an assist device is limited. However, many centres are offering CR programmes for such patients, and the evidence shows that ET can be performed safely. In CRT patients, ET can almost double the improvement in exercise capacity after CRT implantation and further improve haemodynamic parameters and HRQol [13,14].

ICD/CRT patients

The potential benefits of ET for these patients are:

a) familiarization with the device
b) instruction about PA
c) psychological support
d) improvement of exercise capacity.

Nevertheless, several aspects in relation to these patients warrant attention. In order to define exercise duration and interruption criteria correctly, anticipate potential problems, and handle emergencies (instructions for the medical staff), the exercise stress test (EST) in patients with devices needs careful preparation, and the following information should be known:

a) patient history and underlying heart disease
b) arrhythmic substrate or triggers of arrhythmia (ischaemia, HR at onset of ventricular arrhythmia, etc.)
c) indications for device implantation—cardiac arrest, haemodynamic relevant ventricular tachycardia, syncope related to life-threatening ventricular arrhythmia, syncope related to life-threatening ventricular arrhythmia or prophylactic indication (reduced EF) and/or terminal heart disease
d) intervention cut-off point and sequence of therapy (monitoring zone, anti-tachycardia pacing or shocks).

In patients with ICD/CRTs, the information required before an EST goes beyond the diagnosis of ischaemia or the determination of exercise capacity. The following are particularly important:

a) the chronotropic response to exercise
b) the presence of exercise-induced arrhythmias
c) HR in case of the onset of an arrhythmia
d) the effectiveness of pharmacological HR control
e) the risk of reaching an HR in the ICD intervention zone—exercise interruption 10–20 beats below the intervention cut-off required
f) reassurance of the patient and the physician.

In general, ICD patients should start ET under medical supervision. HR should be monitored in order to check whether the protocol brings it near the device's programmed intervention zone. Patients who have experienced symptomatic arrhythmias or ICD discharges should be directed towards exercise modalities in which a short loss of consciousness due to ICD discharge might be less harmful; for example, avoiding strenuous swimming or climbing walls. If there is any intervention by the device, the causes should be assessed and changes in device programming, medication, or exercise regime should be considered. Exercise should be restarted rapidly after device interrogation to avoid the ICD discharge becoming a psychological block on future activity.

Ventricular assist device patients

Although only small study populations limit the evidence regarding the role of ET in VAD patients, all data obtained support the feasibility, safety, and potential benefit [15]. Particular aspects of ET in VAD patients are:

a) requirement for local expertise

b) individual patient factors (e.g. timing of referral, type of intervention delivered, multidisciplinary approach)

c) characteristics of the VAD patients (e.g. combined versus single surgical interventions, type of device, indications for implantation, underlying clinical condition, comorbidities)

d) availability of national recommendations.

Healthcare providers should be familiar not only with exercise physiology and the different exercise modalities but also with device functioning in order to be able to deal with potential complications promptly.

Box 9.2 provides some information about the specific knowledge needed before working with these patients. Vital signs, self-reported symptom scores, and VAD function should be monitored, including the mean arterial pressure in patients on non-pulsatile VAD support because HTN would affect the VAD capacity to pump blood forward. Hypotension and VAD blood flow alterations might be related to under-filling of the left ventricle secondary to high pump speed, RV failure, arrhythmias, etc. The VAD team should be consulted if the mean arterial pressure is below 70mmHg or higher than 90 mmHg, especially when accompanied by VAD alarm

---

Box 9.2 Instructions for reducing the risk of adverse events during ET with VAD patients

- Individualized assessment and prescription.
- Prolonged graduated warm-up and cool-down.
- Low- to moderate-intensity ET.
- Avoid breath-holding and Valsalva manoeuvre.
- Secure of cannulas, drivelines, and the external VAD equipment to prevent damage during mobility.
- Avoid any trauma, as VAD patients are anticoagulated and some (not all) are treated with antiplatelet drugs.
- Monitoring and supervision.
- Keep the patient's feet moving during active recovery if appropriate to allow venous return.
- Observe patients for 15 min after cessation of exercise.

Reproduced from Adamopoulos S, Corra U, Laoutaris ID, et al. Exercise training in patients with ventricular assist devices: a review of the evidence and practical advice. A position paper from the Committee on Exercise Physiology and Training and the Committee of Advanced Heart Failure of the Heart Failure Association of the European Society of Cardiology. *Eur J Heart Fail* 2019;21:3-13, with permission from John Wiley & Sons.

activation. It is also important that the patient is well informed, reassured and feels safe and secure.

Complications related to VAD which may occur are as follows.

a) Drop in LVAD flow or suction alarm.

b) Complex and frequent ventricular arrhythmias on exertion (NB: may be asymptomatic).

c) Infection, mainly at the driveline site: infection control procedures (e.g. cleaning equipment, handwashing, disposal of sharps) should be followed at all times.

d) Evidence of bleeding as VAD patients are anticoagulated or treated with antiplatelet drugs.

e) Thrombus (usually indicated by an increase in the energy (number of watts) necessary to keep the device working).

f) Disconnection from the VAD external power supply.

There are no guidelines describing the specific ET setting, modality, and duration for VAD-supported patients. However, EM should be considered as soon as the patient's haemodynamic and clinical status is stable.

A symptom-limited CPET or 6 min walk test (6-MWT) is advisable for optimizing the workload prescription. If the patient has a peak VO_2 >14 mL/kg/min or a 6-MWT distance >300 m, a more intensive exercise test can be considered.

The following dynamic and resistance exercises are indicated: treadmill (increase ramp, not speed), static bicycle, hamstring curls in standing position, leg press, bicep curls, core stability, respiratory muscle training, and arm ergometry.

Because these patients depend on venous return, it is important to start each ET session with a warm-up phase and to finish with a cool-down phase. Some exercise activities exert torsion on the driveline and therefore must be avoided. Additionally, care should be taken to avoid excessive sweating and dehydration, as well as rapid changes of posture from supine to upright positions, which could reduce venous return and negatively impact VAD function.

Monitoring the exercise sessions is crucial, at least initially, and should include supervision of the patient, clinical adaptation, and VAD functioning [17]. Contraindicated exercises include running, rowing machine, cross trainer, abdominal exercises, bilateral arms above the head with weights or abduction with weights, and swimming.

Conclusion

'High risk' patients are amongst those who profit most from a structured CR programme. However, it is essential to estimate the potential risk of complications in these patients. This implies a thorough clinical assessment, measurement of the haemodynamic and ventilatory response to a functional stress test, and the use of complementary technical examinations when needed. Particular attention must be paid to patients with devices, particularly in conjunction with stress tests and ET, and staff should be given specific instructions regarding this.

References

1. Vanhees L, Rauch B, Piepoli M, et al. Importance of characteristics and modalities of physical activity and exercise in the management of cardiovascular health in individuals with cardiovascular disease (Part III). *Eur J Prev Cardiol* 2012; 19: 1333–56.

2. Piepoli MF, Conraads V, Corrà U, et al. Exercise training in heart failure: from theory to practice. A consensus document of the Heart Failure Association and the European Association for Cardiovascular Prevention and Rehabilitation. *Eur J Heart Fail* 2011; 13: 347–57.

3. Guazzi M, Adams V, Conraads V, et al. EACPR/AHA Joint Scientific Statement. Clinical recommendations for cardiopulmonary exercise testing data assessment in specific patient populations. *Eur Heart J* 2012; 33: 2917–27.

4. Binder RK, Wonisch M, Corrà U, et al. Methodological approach to the first and second lactate threshold in incremental cardiopulmonary exercise testing. *Eur J Cardiovasc Prev Rehabil* 2008; 15: 726–34.

5. Wisloff U, Stoylen A, Loennechen JP, et al. Superior cardiovascular effect of aerobic interval training versus moderate continuous training in heart failure patients: a randomized study. *Circulation* 2007; 115: 3086–94.

6. Ellingsen O, Halle M, Conraads V, et al. High-intensity interval training in patients with heart failure with reduced ejection fraction. *Circulation* 2017; 135:839–49.

7. Guazzi M. High intensity exercise training in heart failure: understanding the exercise 'overdose'. *Eur J Prev Cardiol* 2016; 23: 1940–2.

8. Laoutaris ID. The 'aerobic/resistance/inspiratory muscle training hypothesis in heart failure'. *Eur J Prev Cardiol* 2018; 25: 1257–62.

9. Spruit MA, Eterman RM, Hellwig VA, et al. Effects of moderate-to-high intensity resistance training in patients with chronic heart failure. *Heart* 2009; 95: 1399–1408.

10. Williams MA, Haskell WL, Ades PA, et al. Resistance exercise in individuals with and without cardiovascular disease: 2007 update: a scientific statement from the American Heart Association Council on Clinical Cardiology and Council on Nutrition, Physical Activity, and Metabolism. *Circulation* 2007; 116: 572–84.

11. Ribeiro JP, Chiappa GR, Neder JA, and Frankenstein L. Respiratory muscle function and exercise intolerance in heart failure. *Curr Heart Fail Rep* 2009; 6: 95–101.

12. Laoutaris I, Dritsas A, Brown MD, et al. Inspiratory muscle training using an incremental endurance test alleviates dyspnea and improves functional status in patients with chronic heart failure. *Eur J Cardiovasc Prev Rehabil* 2004; 11: 489–96.

13. Conraads VM, Vanderheyden M, Paelinck B, et al. The effect of endurance training on exercise capacity following cardiac resynchronization therapy in chronic heart failure patients: a pilot trial. *Eur J Cardiovasc Prev Rehabil* 2007; 14: 99–106.

14. Piepoli MF, Villani GQ, Corrà U, et al. Time course of effects of cardiac resynchronization therapy in chronic heart failure: benefits in patients with preserved exercise capacity. *Pacing Clin Electrophysiol* 2008; 31: 701–8.

15. Mahfood Haddad T, Saurav A, Smer A, et al. Cardiac rehabilitation in patients with left ventricular assist device: a systematic review and meta-analysis. *J Cardiopulm Rehabil Prev* 2017; 37: 390–6.

16. Adamopoulos S, Corrà U, et al. Exercise training in patients with ventricular assist devices: a review of the evidence and practical advice. a position paper from the Committee on Exercise Physiology and Training and the Committee of Advanced Heart Failure of the Heart Failure Association of the European Society of Cardiology. *Eur J Heart Fail* 2019; 21: 3–13.

17. Wells CL. Physical therapist management of patients with ventricular assist devices: key considerations for the acute care physical therapist. *Phys Ther* 2013; 93: 266–78.

Further reading

Leggio M, Fusco A, Loreti C, et al. Effects of exercise training in heart failure with preserved ejection fraction: an updated systematic literature review. *Heart Fail Rev* 2019: doi: 10.1007/s10741-019-09841-x.

Severin R, Sabbahi A, Ozemek C, et al. Approaches to improving exercise capacity in patients with left ventricular assist devices: an area requiring further investigation. *Expert Rev Med Devices* 2019; 16: 787–98.

Chapter 10

Diet and nutritional aspects of cardiac rehabilitation

Aimilia Varela, Constantinos H. Davos, and Wolfram Doehner

Summary

Cardiac rehabilitation (CR) and prevention programmes aim to reduce total mortality and rehospitalization and increase health-related quality of life (HRQLI) by supporting behavioural changes such as healthier food habits. Nutritional studies have shown that an approach paying equal attention to what is consumed and what is excluded is more effective in preventing cardiovascular disease (CVD). Mediterranean and dietary approaches to stop hypertension (DASH) diets are the best studied dietary patterns. Both improve a variety of risk features and are associated with lower risk of clinical events in secondary prevention. Patients with acute coronary syndrome (ACS) may respond positively to simple dietary advices, whereas critically ill patients should be appropriately supported in order to reduce the risk of malnutrition and early death. Body weight management in patients with established CVD should be adjusted to individual conditions, risk factors (RFs), and comorbidities, and should be clearly distinguished from simple primary prevention strategies. Unintentional weight loss should be avoided, as an association with increased disease burden, frailty, and adverse outcome has been confirmed. Future studies should focus on the development of specific nutritional guidelines for these patients.

Introduction

CVD prevention through diet and more efficient nutritional choices aims to reduce morbidity and mortality, improve quality of life, and decrease healthcare costs. CR and secondary prevention programmes have been increasingly recommended for patients with chronic CVD and after acute cardiovascular events [1], and meta-analyses of randomized controlled trials (RCTs) show that structured care is associated with better outcomes than standard care. EUROASPIRE IV and V revealed that a large majority of coronary patients in Europe fail to achieve the therapeutic targets of these programmes. These results accord with earlier secondary prevention surveys which show that there are numerous reasons for poor lifestyle adherence, including exercise and healthier food habits, even after a short period post-ACS [2].

As demonstrated by the ONTARGET and TRANSCEND trials, the Nurses' Health Study, and the Health Professional Follow-Up Study, a healthy high-quality diet is associated with a lower risk of all-cause mortality. Thus it is crucial to address dietary habits immediately after hospital discharge, ideally as part of an exercise-based outpatient programme. CR programmes have become multidisciplinary, encompassing exercise training, RF management, psychosocial support, and nutritional counselling in addition to the appropriate use of cardioprotective medication [3].

Diet and nutritional aspects in patients with cardiovascular disease

A cardioprotective diet is characterized not only by specific items to be avoided, but also by healthy foods which are included. Its impact can be evaluated by considering three nutritional parameters:

a) specific nutrients
b) specific foods/food groups
c) specific dietary patterns.

Another important issue is food processing (e.g. cooking, smoking, drying, salting, preserving, etc.) which is also receiving increasing attention. Potential harm includes the loss of food nutrients and the appearance of harmful ingredients such as sodium, trans-fats, heterocyclic amines, advanced glycation end-products etc. [4]. Nutritional counselling has to include estimating individual total daily caloric intake and dietary content of fat, saturated fat, cholesterol, sodium, and other nutrients, assessing eating habits (number of meals, frequency of dining out, alcohol consumption), and assessing target areas for nutritional interventions (body weight, dyslipidaemia, arterial hypertension, diabetes mellitus (DM), heart failure, and other comorbidities [5]. Table 10.1 shows the general principles of healthy diet [6–8].

A palaeolithic diet, which is a plant-based diet including fruit, nuts, vegetables, fish, and lean meat, and is low in grains, sugar, and salt, has also been proposed. Although several clinical studies report beneficial effects on CV and other metabolic risk biomarkers, few studies have explored the association of a paleolithic diet pattern with chronic disease endpoints. However, although a paleolithic diet has favourable effects on CVD RFs, the evidence is not conclusive and more well-designed trials are required [9].

Another diet pattern focuses on ketone-providing nutrients, but more studies are required to establish the long-term effects of this diet on CVD RFs and better define which dietary macronutrient composition is optimal or acceptable for ACS patients. These diets are generally high in fats and/or proteins and very low in carbohydrates. According to the American Diabetes Association, the standard composition of a ketogenic diet in adults supplying 2000 kcal/day is defined as <130 g carbohydrate per day or <26% of caloric intake. It seems that the most significant effects (improvements in CVD RFs such as obesity, type 2 DM, and high-density lipid (HDL)

Table 10.1 General principles of a healthy diet
1. Saturated fatty acids (<10% of total energy intake)
2. Trans unsaturated fatty acids: no intake from processed food and <1% of total energy intake from natural origin
3. <5–6 g of salt per day
4. 30–45 g of fibre per day preferably from whole grain products
5. 200 g of fruit per day (2–3 servings)
6. 200 g of vegetables per day (2–3 servings)
7. Extra virgin olive oil, tea, cocoa, and soya (rich in polyphenols)
8. Fish at least three times per week, including two servings of oily fish
9. Foods rich in fibre
10. Red meat (beef once or twice per week, mutton/lamb once a month) and cooked meats to 70–100 g per week
11. Butter replacement with a margarine rich in omega-3 fatty acids
12. Eggs restricted to 4–6 per week
13. Cheese restricted to 30–40 g per day
14. Alcoholic consumption should be limited to two glasses per day (alcohol, 20 g/day) for men and one glass per day (alcohol, 10 g/day) for women

Source data from Trichopoulou A, Bamia C, Norat T, et al. Modified Mediterranean diet and survival aer myocardial infarction: the EPIC-Elderly study. *Eur J Epidemiol* 2007;22(12):871-81.

Piepoli MF, Villani GQ. Lifestyle modification in secondary prevention. *Eur J Prev Cardiol* 2017;24(3_ suppl):101-107. doi: 10.1177/2047487317703828.

Chiavaroli L, Viguiliouk E, Nishi SK, et al. DASH Dietary Pattern and Cardiometabolic Outcomes: An Umbrella Review of Systematic Reviews and Meta-Analyses. *Nutrients* 2019;11(2). pii: E338. doi: 10.3390/nu11020338.

cholesterol levels) are due to the reduced caloric intake and an increased satiety effect of proteins. The duration of a ketogenic diet may range from 2–3 weeks to a maximum of many months (6–12 months). Attention should be paid to patient's renal function and the transition from the ketogenic to the normal pattern which has to be gradual [10].

Recommendations on adequate caloric intake should take the individual's status and activity level into consideration. A negative caloric balance should be avoided, except when weight reduction is intended, but this should be advised with great care as acute and chronic CVD are often characterized by catabolic dominance, with loss of muscle (sarcopenia) and total body weight (cachexia) being signs of disease progression and worse outcome. There are no specific recommendations related to the percentage of energy substrates that must be included. Provision of essential amino acids is necessary in the critically ill. Evidence suggests that 1.2–1.5 g/kg/day of protein is needed [11–13]. The kcal/g N_2 ratio should be maintained at 100–150:1; decreasing it is based on the degree of protein depletion or the increase in metabolic stress. Carbohydrates should not exceed 6 g/kg/day and lipids should not exceed 2.5 g/kg/day.

Accounting for comorbidities, diabetes mellitus, and hypertension

Exercise is likely to induce specific metabolic benefits in patients with DM. Blood glucose should repeatedly be checked before, at the end of the exercise, and 4–6 h after an exercise session or physical activity (PA) in every patient with DM to reduce the risk of hypoglycaemic episodes. A balance between ingested carbohydrates and insulin is critical for post-prandial blood glucose control. For prevention of CAD, it is recommended that saturated fats are reduced to <10% of total energy intake (if possible, to <7%), trans-fatty acids should be avoided. A Mediterranean-style diet rich in fruit, vegetables, and mono-unsaturated fatty acids is also recommended [14].

Hypertension management should include exercise training, weight management, sodium restriction, alcohol moderation, and smoking cessation. Lipid management should include a detailed history to determine whether diet, drug use, and/or other conditions that might affect lipid levels could be altered, assess current treatment and compliance, provide nutritional counselling and weight management, increase HDL to at least 35 mg/dL, advise exercise training and smoking cessation, and consider drug therapy to achieve guideline targets. Patients are generally encouraged to adopt a complex-carbohydrate lower-fat diet that emphasizes consumption of whole grains, fruit, and vegetables [15].

Nutritional aspects in patients with malnutrition issues

Patients with CVD may develop overlapping types of malnutrition: cardiac cachexia (which is a global wasting of body tissues in all compartments) or sarcopenia (specific wasting of muscle tissue). Early enteral nutrition should be attempted if the oral route cannot be used.

Critically ill cardiac syndromes include the following: ACS, decompensated chronic heart failure (HF), chronic systemic inflammatory response syndrome, cardiac surgery, and patients with acute heart disease such as development of complications from another condition (chronic systemic inflammatory response syndrome, sepsis, etc.). Enteral nutrition could be indicated if complications occur [12]. Nutritional assessment aims to identify baseline nutritional status and risk of malnutrition, and to develop a diet care plan to prevent unintended weight loss and monitor its efficacy. Changing the metabolic setting from catabolic to anabolic, reducing free-radical production, and decreasing inflammation levels, in addition to caloric supplementation, may be the key targets for nutritional support in HF patients [11].

It has been shown that patients with CVD may respond positively to simple dietary advice, and this may contribute to a substantial reduction in the risk of early death. Regardless of any drug treatment, clinicians should routinely advise ACS patients to adhere to a Mediterranean diet as it reduces the risk of premature death after a heart attack [16]. The association between this diet and CAD may be attributable to the protective effect of its components which contain nutrients with anti-oxidant and anti-inflammatory action, including omega-3 fatty acids, oleic acid, vitamins B6, B12,

C and E, folic acid, and phenolic compounds, as well as fibre. However, none of these foods shows a dominant effect. Recently, the PREDIMED and the CARDIO2000 trials reported that a Mediterranean diet supplemented with olive oil decreases the likelihood of an ACS event and reduces mortality in high-risk patients [17]. It has been demonstrated that patients with a recent myocardial infarction (within the previous three months) who follow a daily 30 min supervised aerobic exercise session should also adopt a Mediterranean style diet (more bread, fruit, vegetables, and fish, less meat, and replacement of butter and cream with rapeseed margarine) [18].

Another study has revealed that the addition of a cardioprotective diet to PA as a part of a CR programme positively modifies not just classic RFs (i.e. body mass index (BMI), waist circumference, systolic BP, blood glucose, and low-density lipoprotein (LDL) cholesterol) and exercise capacity (maximal work load, maximal exercise time), but also diminishes chronic inflammation markers (high-sensitivity C-reactive protein, interleukin-6, oxidative LDL). This PA programme included daily interval ergometric training, stretching, and respiratory exercises. Each patient from the diet group had a meeting with a clinical dietician who assembled an individual menu according to their weight, body composition, presence of DM, and personal preferences. The percentage of macronutrients depended on individual needs, but in general the diet was composed of 25% fat, 60% carbohydrates, and 15% proteins. Patients with DM had a lower percentage of carbohydrates and a higher percentage of proteins [19]. Further, patients with moderate to severe CAD may benefit from a low-fat vegetarian diet for at least a year in parallel with an exercise programme such as 30 min walking every day or at least 3 hours per week, with reduction in cardiovascular mortality and non-fatal cardiovascular events [20]. This type of diet includes fruit, vegetables, grains, and soybean products, with no animal products except egg white and one cup of non-fat milk or yoghurt daily.

Hyperglycaemia should be closely monitored, and hyperglycaemic peaks should be avoided similarly to hypoglycaemia episodes secondary to PA, although the latter may pose a higher risk of acute complications. Administration of carnitine (3–6 g in divided doses) may lead to improved haemodynamic status and myocardial dysfunction, and glutamine may be beneficial for patients with myocardial ischaemia in a critical situation. It is recommended that at least 1 g/day omega-3 (EPA + DHA) and supplements containing vitamins A, C, B complex, E, and D, calcium, magnesium, zinc, and selenium should be administered to patients with ACS who require enteral nutrition. Parenteral nutrition is indicated for cardiac cachexia if there is intolerance to enteral nutrition or as complementary nutrition [21].

Weight management and risk of cachexia and frailty

Cachexia has traditionally been viewed as a condition of severe weight loss in late-stage chronic disease, but there is current evidence that there is already a detrimental impact on disease progression, poor HRQoL, and mortality with a comparatively small but measurable degree of weight loss. Accordingly, cachexia is defined as an unintentional weight loss of 5% body weight within 12 months accompanied by three of the following five criteria: decreased muscle strength, fatigue, anorexia, low fat mass index, or abnormal biochemical results of inflammatory and metabolic blood tests [22]. Notably, this degree of weight loss has been associated with increased mortality independent of the starting point of BMI and also applies to overweight or mildly obese subjects. In turn, overweight and mild obesity are related to lower mortality as shown by multiple observations (Figure 10.1) [23,24]. While prevention of excessive body weight is a well-established principle in the primary prevention of cardiovascular diseases, evidence from RCTs of a benefit of weight reduction in the presence of cardiovascular disease is lacking. The LOOK AHEAD study of 5145 patients with established DM investigated whether a prospective comprehensive weight reduction programme would translate into clinical and outcome benefit [25]. The controlled trial did not show a benefit from the achieved weight reduction for any clinical outcome (mortality, cardiovascular events). Therefore weight reduction recommendations should be advocated with great caution, based on the individual patient's characteristics and comorbidities. A mere translation of primary

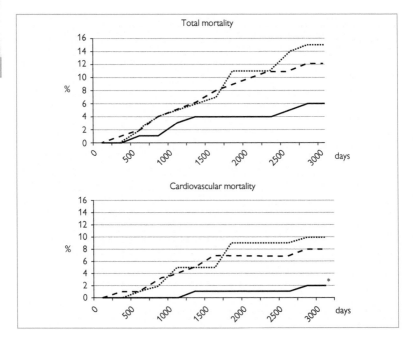

Figure 10.1 BMI and mortality in CR. The study included 389 patients during CR (mean follow-up 6.4±1.8 years). Normal weight, BMI 18.5–25 kg/m²; overweight, BMI >25–30 kg/m²; obese, BMI >30 kg/m².

*p <0.05, adjusted for age and gender.

Reproduced from Sierra-Johnson J, Wright SR, Lopez-Jimenez F, Allison TG. Relation of body mass index to fatal and nonfatal cardiovascular events after cardiac rehabilitation. Am J Cardiol 2005; 96(2): 211–14. doi:10.1016/j.amjcard.2005.03.046 with permission from Elsevier.

prevention evidence for body weight management to patients with established CVD does not seem to be advisable.

Consultations regarding nutrition, lifestyle, and inflammation should be based on the information in Table 10.2 [26].

Nutrition is a very important part of the multidimensional intervention in CR, particularly in very elderly and frail or sarcopenic/cachectic patients, where poor nutritional status is one of the main pathophysiological mechanisms of frailty [27]. Recent studies suggest that improving nutritional status may reduce the risk of frailty [28]. Nutrition and exercise interventions (resistance training, aerobic exercises, and flexibility and balance exercises) can increase muscle strength and/or mass, and improve in physical performance. Dietary strategies include dietary supplementation and increased intakes of a range of high-quality nutrients and bioactive non-nutrients. Nutritional supplements usually include protein or amino acid supplementation, multi-nutrient supplementation, and vitamin D or creatine supplementation. Supplementation may include 7–20 g protein, 10–40 g carbohydrates, and 1 g fat (169 kcal) consumed either before or immediately after exercise [29]. Total protein intake appears to be significantly inversely associated with frailty in elderly patients, and this is observed regardless of the protein source or its amino acid composition.

Table 10.2 Nutrition, lifestyle, and inflammation	
Pro-inflammatory factors (to be avoided)	Anti-inflammatory factors (should be preferred)
Sugars	Oily fish and fish oil supplements
Saturated fats	Olives and olive oil
Excess alcohol	Walnut or flaxseed oil
Sedentary lifestyle	Fruit and vegetables
Periodontal or gum disease	Nuts or zinc tablets
Trans-fats found in partially hydrogenated oils (margarine, vegetable shortening)	Garlic, ginger, turmeric (curcumin), sunflower seeds
	Omega-3 fatty acid supplements
	Pineapple or bromelain supplements
	Grapefruit juice
	Red wine (small amounts)
	Antioxidant supplements (vitamins C and E)
	S-adenosyl-methionine
	Alpha-lipoic acid
	Coenzyme Q10
	Abdominal fat reduction, stress reduction, teeth flossing

Conclusion

Nutrition largely determines our health status. Therefore, dietary guidelines have been developed to guide nutritional recommendations for healthy dietary habits aimed at preventing or delaying the onset of age-related disease (primary prevention) and reducing the risks in patients with already established disease (secondary outcome prevention). However, these global recommendations cannot address the individual needs and preferences driven by comorbidities, genetic, and cultural factors [30]. The status, risk profiles, and modifiable and non-modifiable factors of individual patients need to be taken into consideration in order to achieve appropriate personalized nutritional and/or weight management recommendations. The response to a dietary intervention may vary considerably among individuals, with no benefit in some and substantial benefit in others [31].

Despite the favourable association between healthy diet and a reduced risk of CAD, maintaining dietary changes in daily life is challenging. The dynamics of dietary factors and CAD progression are complex and multifactorial. Thus further efforts are needed to support long-term adherence to dietary recommendations,. According to the most recent ESC guidelines, the future challenge is to translate nutritional guidelines into attractive diets and to find ways to make people change their long-standing dietary habits.

References

1. Perk J, Hambraeus K, Burell G, et al. Study of Patient Information after percutaneous Coronary Intervention (SPICI): should prevention programmes become more effective? *EuroIntervention* 2015; 10(11): e1–7.

2. Kotseva K, De Backer G, De Bacquer D, et al. Lifestyle and impact on cardiovascular risk factor control in coronary patients across 27 countries: results from the European Society of Cardiology ESC-EORP EUROASPIRE V registry. *Eur J Prev Cardiol* 2019; 26(8): 824–35.

3. Cole JA, Smith SM, Hart N, Cupples ME. Systematic review of the effect of diet and exercise lifestyle interventions in the secondary prevention of coronary heart disease. *Cardiol Res Pract* 2011; 2011: 232351.

4. Pavy B, Barbet R, Carré F, et al. Therapeutic education in coronary heart disease: position paper from the Working Group of Exercise Rehabilitation and Sport (GERS) and the Therapeutic Education Commission of the French Society of Cardiology. *Arch Cardiovasc Dis* 2013; 106: 680–9.

5. Balady GJ, Ades PA, Comoss P, et al. Core components of cardiac rehabilitation/secondary prevention programs: a statement for healthcare professionals from the American Heart Association and the American Association of Cardiovascular and Pulmonary Rehabilitation Writing Group. *Circulation* 2000; 102: 1069–73.

6. Trichopoulou A, Bamia C, Norat T, et al. Modified Mediterranean diet and survival after myocardial infarction: the EPIC-Elderly study. *Eur J Epidemiol* 2007; 22: 871–81.

7. Piepoli MF, Villani GQ. Lifestyle modification in secondary prevention. *Eur J Prev Cardiol* 2017; 24: 101–7.

8. Chiavaroli L, Viguiliouk E, Nishi SK, et al. DASH dietary pattern and cardiometabolic outcomes: an umbrella review of systematic reviews and meta-analyses. *Nutrients* 2019; 11: 338.

9. Otten J, Stomby A, Waling M, et al. Benefits of a paleolithic diet with and without supervised exercise on fat mass, insulin sensitivity, and glycemic control: a randomized controlled trial in individuals with type 2 diabetes. *Diabetes Metab Res Rev* 2017; 33: doi 10.1002/dmrr.2828.

10. Paoli A. Ketogenic diet for obesity: friend or foe? *Int J Environ Res Public Health* 2014; 11(2): 2092–107.

11. Meltzer JS, Moitra VK. The nutritional and metabolic support of heart failure in the intensive care unit. *Curr Opin Clin Nutr Metab Care* 2008; 11: 140–6.

12. Jiménez Jiménez FJ, Cervera Montes M, Blesa Malpica AL, et al. Guidelines for specialized nutritional and metabolic support in the critically-ill patient: update. Consensus SEMICYUC-SENPE: cardiac patient. *Nutr Hosp* 2011; 26(Suppl 2): 76–80.

13. Hill A, Nesterova E, Lomivorotov V, et al. Current evidence about nutrition support in cardiac surgery patients.What do we know? *Nutrients* 2018; 10: E597. doi: 10 3390/nu10050597

14. Vergès B, Avignon A, Bonnet F, et al. Consensus statement on the care of the hyperglycaemic/diabetic patient during and in the immediate follow-up of acute coronary syndrome. *Arch Cardiovasc Dis* 2012; 105: 239–53.

15. Ades PA, Savage PD, Harvey-Berino J. The treatment of obesity in cardiac rehabilitation. *J Cardiopulm Rehabil Prev* 2010; 30: 289–98.

16. Barzi F, Woodward M, Marfisi RM, et al. Mediterranean diet and all-causes mortality after myocardial infarction: results from the GISSI-Prevenzione trial. *Eur J Clin Nutr* 2003; 57: 604–11.

17. Kouvari M, Notara V, Panagiotakos DB,et al. Exclusive olive oil consumption and 10-year (2004–2014) acute coronary syndrome incidence among cardiac patients: the GREECS observational study. *J Hum Nutr Diet* 2016; 29: 354–62.

18. Skinner JS, Cooper A. Secondary prevention of ischaemic cardiac events. *BMJ Clin Evid* 2011; 2011: 0206.

19. Mlakar P, Salobir B, Čobo N, et al. The effect of cardioprotective diet rich with natural antioxidants on chronicinflammation and oxidized LDL during cardiac rehabilitation in patients after acute myocardial infarction. *Int J Cardiol Heart Vasc* 2015; 7: 40–8.

20. Ornish D, Scherwitz LW, Billings JH, et al. Intensive lifestyle changes for reversal of coronary heart disease. *JAMA* 1998; 280: 2001–7. Erratum: *JAMA* 1999 21; 281: 1380.

21. Preiser JC, van Zanten AR, Berger MM, et al. Metabolic and nutritional support of critically ill patients: consensus and controversies. *Crit Care* 2015; 19: 35.

22. Evans WJ, Morley JE, Argilés J, et al. Cachexia: a new definition. *Clin Nutr* 2008; 27: 793–9.

23. Sierra-Johnson J, Wright SR, Lopez-Jimenez F, Allison TG. Relation of body mass index to fatal and nonfatal cardiovascular events after cardiac rehabilitation. *Am J Cardiol* 2005; 96: 211–14.

24. Doehner W, von Haehling S, Anker SD. Protective overweight in cardiovascular disease: moving from 'paradox' to 'paradigm'. *Eur Heart J* 2015; 36: 2729–32.

25. LOOK AHEAD Research Group. Cardiovascular effects of intensive lifestyle intervention in type 2 diabetes. *N Engl J Med* 2013; 369: 145–54

26. Azhar G, Wei JY. Nutrition and cardiac cachexia. *Curr Opin Clin Nutr Metab Care* 2006; 9: 18–23.

27. Morley JE, Vellas B, van Kan GA, et al. Frailty consensus: a call to action: *J Am Med Dir Assoc* 2013; 14: 392–7.

28. Vigorito C, Abreu A, Ambrosetti M, et al. Frailty and cardiac rehabilitation: a call to action from the EAPC Cardiac Rehabilitation Section. *Eur J Prev Cardiol* 2017; 24: 577–90.

29. Denison HJ, Cooper C, Sayer AA, Robinson SM. Prevention and optimal management of sarcopenia: a review of combined exercise and nutrition interventions to improve muscle outcomes in older people. *Clin Interv Aging.* 2015; 10: 859–69.

30. Konstantinidou V, Daimiel L, Ordovás JM. Personalized nutrition and cardiovascular disease prevention: from Framingham to PREDIMED. *Adv Nutr* 2014; 5 :368S–71S.

31. Lacroix S, Cantin J, Nigam A. Contemporary issues regarding nutrition in cardiovascular rehabilitation. *Ann Phys Rehabil Med* 2017; 60: 36–42.

Chapter 11

Educational intervention

Marie Christine Iliou and Margaret E. Cupples

Summary

The impact of a cardiac disease diagnosis on patients is multidimensional. Educational interventions are at the core of the delivery of effective therapy and require multidisciplinary teamwork to identify specific impacts on individuals and coordinate activities to support changes in lifestyle behaviour. Motivational interviewing and negotiation, based on a comprehensive assessment of patients' circumstances, should identify the support they require to engage in preventive programmes. Interventions to help patients to apply new knowledge to their everyday lives should be underpinned by the use of recognized educational principles to optimize their adoption of new behaviours. Meaningful communication between professionals and patients must be timely and ongoing, to allow appropriate feedback on progress and revision of forward plans for optimal cardiac rehabilitation (CR) and secondary prevention. The quality of programmes delivered should be evaluated regularly using specified criteria.

Introduction

Patient education refers to the process by which information is given to patients by health professionals and others, aiming to change their health behaviours or improve their health status. Patient education includes both prevention and health promotion and, in facilitating behaviour change, plays a key role in cardiac disease management.

Education is a core element of CR and secondary prevention [1]. However, although information increases knowledge and can influence behaviour, it alone may be insufficient to ensure behaviour change. In clinical practice, awareness of lifestyle factors is important, and empathetic counselling and advice are needed to support patients in applying knowledge to their lives. An educational intervention for patients with cardiovascular disease (CVD) must incorporate a structured plan which includes evaluation, negotiation, and application.

General considerations

In addition to the pathophysiological impact, CVD can have significant emotional, psychological, and social impact on patients, their families, and their friends. Thus, interventions for these patients should be provided by a multidisciplinary team, including doctors, nurses, physiotherapists, dieticians, social workers, and psychologists. Although based on limited evidence, a recent Cochrane Review [2] concluded that educational interventions should be included in comprehensive CR programmes with exercise and psychological support. Principles of patient education should be integral in every patient–doctor encounter for effective secondary prevention across the lifespan.

Therapeutic patient education [3] fundamentally and sustainably changes the values and roles of caregivers and encourages involvement of new healthcare actors such as patient associations. Its ultimate purpose is, through caregivers and patients working in partnership, to obtain a therapeutic alliance and change the posture of the patient from that of a spectator (who listens, hears, obeys, follows instructions) to that of a protagonist in the care system (gives an opinion, negotiates, adapts instructions, understands). For this, the patient must acquire knowledge as well as expertise in self-care and the skills needed to adapt to lifestyle change.

Key practical points within an educational programme to provide optimal support for patients in CR and secondary prevention are as follows.

a) Establish a precise diagnosis, inform the patient, and ensure that they understand (check how they would tell someone else) its causes, risk factors, treatment/medication (including side effects), and signs/symptoms that should alert them to contact a physician.

b) Identify the programme's objectives (from perspectives of caregivers and patients).

c) Establish a shared educational needs assessment, including physical, emotional, and social considerations and health literacy, updated regularly as the programme progresses.

d) Develop realistic achievable operational goals in partnership with the patient.

e) Establish an individualized, progressive plan of action, respecting the patient's capabilities, opportunities, and motivation.

f) Identify, in partnership with the patient, the psychosocial and practical support needed to implement the plan.

g) Agree how to monitor progress towards goals (e.g. blood biochemistry, weight, smoking habit, physical activity (PA), diet, well-being/HrQOL, diary record, questionnaires).

h) Assess progress: review monitoring data, provide feedback on progress, discuss possible constraints and fears, and review choice of goals and programme objectives.

i) Reformulate the educational programme and management plan as appropriate.

These issues should be considered by healthcare professionals during every encounter with patients with cardiac disease. More practical details of specific educational interventions are discussed in the following sections.

Evaluation and motivational interview

In order to develop a relevant education programme, the multidisciplinary team needs to know about various aspects of the patient's life, not only their diagnosis (bioclinical dimension) but also their everyday activities within their occupation, family, and community responsibilities and leisure time (social dimension). It is also important to assess their knowledge and understanding of their diagnosis and treatment (cognitive dimension), their personality (psychological dimension), and their forward plan (willingness to adopt secondary prevention recommendations, including medication).

A motivational interview [4] aims to increase the patient's intrinsic motivation to change, by exploring their ambivalence and resolve, and supporting them in developing an appreciation of the value of possible changes in their lifestyle behaviour. For this, the health professional must help the patient to explore the reasoning that determines their attitude to change and their resistance to or acceptance of recommendations. All aspects of the patient's lifestyle and personality (positive and negative) should be considered, including CV risk factors, behaviour before the cardiac event, level of cognition, sociocultural and physical environment, and barriers and obstacles to behaviour change. The professional must work collaboratively with the patient to achieve concordance in planning, avoiding confrontation and persuasion, favouring open questions, showing an empathetic attitude, and being prepared to revise plans in future encounters.

Trading/negotiation

The patient's clinical status and information gained through motivational interviewing will inform the content of an educational programme and holistic management plan, negotiated between the health professional and patient. Negotiation must include consideration of personal safety, awareness of signs/symptoms of need for medical help, the contributions of the multidisciplinary team and of the patient, and the resources needed to support lifestyle changes. Clear objectives should be defined, using a SMART acronym: **S**pecific (personalized), **M**easurable (can be evaluated), **A**chievable (possible for the patient), **R**ealistic (applicable to the patient), and **T**emporal (evaluated at a specific time).

Examples of relevant components of negotiations relating to the domains of knowledge, self-care, and adaptation are as follows for two selected conditions:

Chronic coronary syndrome

1. Knowledge: explain diagnosis, specific risk factors, mechanism of action of treatment, including medication and side effects, the value of a Mediterranean diet, and the principles of exercise.
2. Self-care: self-monitoring blood pressure (BP), diet, exercise, smoking, alcohol habits; appropriate action if chest pain occurs; exercise plan, with plans to adapt intensity and frequency.
3. Adaptation skills: management of stress; return to work/social responsibility; incorporate healthy diet and PA in daily life routine; avoid smoking.

Heart failure

1. Knowledge: explain disease cause and trajectory, signs/symptoms of condition worsening, limitations on salt consumption, effects of medication.
2. Self-care: self-monitoring of weight, BP, heart rate; medication; blood markers; appropriate action if worsening dyspnoea or oedema.
3. Adaptation skills: how to adapt daily life to the clinical condition; live within/ adapt physical and social environment.

Educational sessions

Motivational interviewing and negotiation often focus on a particular aspect of behaviour and are usually conducted in one-to-one encounters, but comprehensive educational sessions are core to longer-term management. Trained professionals should conduct these sessions using various models (group or individual sessions, theoretical and/or practical), and cover core components including PA, diet/nutritional and smoking cessation counselling, exercise prescription, weight, lipid, and BP management, and vocational and psychosocial support [1]. Educational approaches may include interactive presentations, such as discussion of hypothetical scenarios (e.g. Mr X after a myocardial infarction takes all his meals at restaurant . . . , forgetting to take medication . . .), visual prompts/photo-language (e.g. about diet or stress), games (e.g. regarding anticoagulant dosages), practical actions (e.g. self-monitoring blood glucose), and skills training (e.g. cooking healthy meals, shopping).

The advantages of group sessions (efficient use of professionals' time, the extent of information provided and exchange of patient experiences, conviviality, and emotional support) generally outweigh those of individual sessions. However, group sessions may have disadvantages, including heterogeneity of patients which may inhibit individuals in discussing their condition, difficulties in group dynamics, and risk of patient conflict.

A typical educational session should include the following: presentation of the session's objective, information about the speaker(s), and duration; introduction of each participant, asking them to share their expectations of the session; information provision, checking baseline knowledge, encouraging discussions, correcting misinformation, and ensuring understanding; synthesizing and revising forward plans for the programme. The efficiency of these sessions may be improved if the moderator is assisted by another professional or an experienced patient.

Each educational session should be evaluated by participants; their feedback should be used to revise and improve the programme's design and delivery. Quality criteria for evaluation of an educational intervention are suggested in Table 11.1.

Table 11.1 Quality criteria for educational intervention in cardiac rehabilitation	
Criteria	Evidence required
Patient-focused	Responsive to individuals' needs
Evidence-based	High-quality studies
Multidisciplinary	Multiprofessional team
Trained healthcare providers	CR training course attendance
Clear information	Lay language; pictorial
Patients understand diagnosis, causes, treatment, management, signs/symptoms	Patients can explain their condition, care plan, when urgent care is needed, points of contact
Assessment of clinical and psychosocial needs; access to services and support	Negotiation of holistic individual care plans
Programme evaluation, ongoing review	Patient satisfaction questionnaire, audit, attendance and achievement of goals
Communication timely, relevant, inclusive	Clear communication pathways for patients and professionals

The frequency and duration of educational programmes vary widely [2]; typically educational sessions are provided at least once weekly over eight weeks, but further evidence is needed to inform optimal programme design [5]. Home-based or telemonitoring follow-up plans may be developed for patients who have difficulty travelling to a centre.

Conclusion

Effective educational interventions in CR require multidisciplinary teamwork to coordinate activities and relay meaningful communications between professionals and patients. Motivational interviewing and negotiation of management plans should be based on a comprehensive assessment of patients' physical and social circumstances which identifies the support required to optimize their engagement in preventive programmes. Recognized educational principles which underpin the design of these interventions facilitate patients' application of knowledge into practice in their everyday lives.

References

1. Piepoli MF, Corrà U, Adamopoulos S, et al. Secondary prevention in the clinical management of patients with cardiovascular diseases. Core components, standards and outcome measures for referral and delivery. A Policy Statement from the Cardiac Rehabilitation Section of the European Association for Cardiovascular Prevention and Rehabilitation. Endorsed by the Committee for Practice Guidelines of the European Society of Cardiology. *Eur J Prev Cardiol* 2014; 21: 664–81.

2. Anderson L, Brown JP, Clark AM, et al. Patient education in the management of coronary heart disease. *Cochrane Database Syst Rev* 2017; 6: CD008895.

3. WHO Regional Office for Europe, Copenhagen. *Therapeutic Patient Education. Continuing Education Programmes for Health Care Providers in the Field of Prevention of Chronic Diseases*. Report of a WHO Working Group, 1998.

4. Rollnick S, Heather N, Bell A. Negotiating behaviour change in medical settings: the development of brief motivational interviewing. *J Ment Health* 1992; 1: 25–37.

5. Piepoli MF, Hoes AW, Agewall S, et al. 2016 European Guidelines on cardiovascular disease prevention in clinical practice. The Sixth Joint Task Force of the European Society of Cardiology and Other Societies on Cardiovascular Disease Prevention in Clinical. *Eur Heart J* 2016; 37: 2315–81.

Further reading

Kabboul NN, Tomlinson G, Francis TA, et al. Comparative effectiveness of the core components of cardiac rehabilitation on mortality and morbidity: a systematic review and network meta-analysis. *J Clin Med* 2018; 7. pii: E514.

Kourbelis CM, Marin TS, Foote J, et al. Effectiveness of discharge education strategies versus usual care on clinical outcomes in acute coronary syndrome patients: a systematic review. *JBI Evid Synth* 2020; 18: 309–31.

Messerli AW, Deutsch C. Implementation of institutional discharge protocols and transition of care following acute coronary syndrome. *Cardiovasc Revasc Med* 2020. pii: S1553-8389(20)30083-X.

Wallert J, Olsson EM, Pingel R, et al. Attending Heart School and long-term outcome after myocardial infarction: a decennial SWEDEHEART registry study. *Eur J Prev Cardiol* 2020; 27: 145–54.

Chapter 12

Intervention for depression, anxiety, and stress in cardiovascular patients

Manuela Abreu

Summary

The strong influence of depression on adherence to treatment and the prognosis of coronary artery disease (CAD) is emphasized in the 2016 European Guidelines on the prevention of cardiovascular disease (CVD) in clinical practice and in the 2019 European Society of Cardiology Guidelines for the diagnosis and management of chronic coronary syndromes. Therefore it is important that health professionals working in cardiac rehabilitation (CR) are aware of (a) the importance of depression on cardiac mortality, (b) the tools for diagnosis, and (c) the principles of treatment and their impact on prognosis in depressed cardiac patients. Treating depression has the potential to improve CV outcomes, and selective serotonin reuptake inhibitors (SSRIs) are the first-line antidepressants in coronary heart disease patients. However, it is essential to educate patients about side effects, to monitor them closely, and to be aware of interactions with other medications.

Introduction

Depression has mainly been assessed in the context of CAD where a bidirectional relationship has been demonstrated. In fact, depression is not only an independent risk factor (RF) for the development of CAD, but also has a significant impact on prognosis [1].

About 15–20% of patients with an acute myocardial infarction (AMI) satisfy the criteria for a major depression episode as defined in the *Diagnostic and Statistical Manual of Mental Disorders* (DSM-5), and many more will present with subsyndromal depressive symptoms.

In patients with coronary artery disease (CAD), both major depression and depressive symptoms increase the risk of fatal and non-fatal cardiac events, as well as the risk of all-cause mortality. In a Scientific Statement published in 2014, the American Heart Association considered depression as a RF for poor prognosis in patients with ACS [2]. The great importance of depression with respect to adherence to treatment and prognosis of CAD is also emphasized in the 2016 European Guidelines on CVD prevention in clinical practice and in the 2019 ESC Guidelines on the diagnosis and management of chronic coronary syndromes. Therefore the most important questions are as follows.

a) How does depression increase cardiac mortality?
b) How is depression in cardiac patients diagnosed?
c) How is depression treated?
d) Does treatment of depression reduce mortality in cardiac patients?

How does depression increase cardiac mortality?

Depression has biological and behavioural consequences that lead to a higher risk of cardiac events and cardiac mortality.

Biological consequences of depression

a) Platelet dysfunction which causes a prothrombotic state.
b) Activation of the hypothalamic–pituitary–adrenal–cortical axis leading to hypercortisolaemia.
c) Sympatho-medullar hyperactivity.
d) Reduced heart rate (HR) variability.
e) Endothelial dysfunction.
f) Activation of inflammation.

Behavioural consequences of depression

A depressed cardiac patient, in a state of anhedonia, with lack of energy and mo-tivation, has an increased risk of poor adherence to treatment as well as missing medical appointments. He will not be motivated to stop smoking, to change his sedentary lifestyle, or to start a healthy diet. The thought of physical exercise or CR is unbearable because his lack of motivation makes him feel as if someone has turned off the energy button. This depressive behaviour increases the risk of fur-ther cardiac events, and our task is to diagnose and promptly treat depression in these patients.

How do we diagnose depression in cardiac patients?

Accordingly to the DSM-5 criteria, patients complain of depressed mood and/or mark-edly diminished interest or pleasure in activities, together with at least five of the fol-lowing symptoms: weight loss or gain (>5%); insomnia or hypersomnia; psychomotor retardation or agitation; fatigue or loss of energy; feelings of worthlessness or guilt; reduced ability to concentrate or think; recurrent thoughts of death [3]. However, de-pressive symptoms in cardiac patients often differ from those observed in psychiatric patients. The clinical depression might not be so obvious, which is why it is called 'masked depression'. Instead of depressed mood, cardiac patient often present with somatic symptoms such as fatigue, reduced ability to concentrate, sleep disorders, and loss of energy. This different clinical presentation of depression is an important factor in under-diagnosing and under-treating depression among cardiac patients.

In order to screen depression in cardiac inpatients, we can use a quick and reliable tool, such as the Patient Health Questionnaire-2 (PHQ-2) [4] which consists of two items:

'Over the past 2 weeks, how often have you been bothered by any of the following problems?'
  (1) Little interest or pleasure in doing things.
  (2) Feeling down, depressed, or hopeless.

If the answer is 'yes' to either question, the patient must respond to PHQ-9, a questionnaire consisting of nine items:

'Over the past 2 weeks, how often have you been bothered by any of the following problems?'
  (1) Little interest or pleasure in doing things
  (2) Feeling down, depressed or hopelessness
  (3) Troubling falling or staying asleep or sleeping too much
  (4) Feeling tired or having little energy
  (5) Poor appetite or overeating
  (6) Feeling bad about yourself or that you are a failure or let yourself or your family down
  (7) Trouble concentrating on things such as reading the newspaper or watching TV
  (8) Moving or speaking so slowly that other people could have noticed—or being restless
  (9) Thoughts that you would be better off dead, or hurting yourself in some way.

Interpretation of results:

a) score 0–27

b) score ≥10 predicts a clinical depression episode

c) sensitivity and specificity 88%.

Other reliable questionnaires often used for evaluation of depression are the Hospital Anxiety and Depression Scale (HADS) and the Beck Depression Inventory (BDI). If patients have high scores on these questionnaires, a psychiatric consultation should be considered with a structured clinical interview and use of other depression rating scales, such as the Hamilton Depression Rating Scale (HAMD) or the Montgomery–Åsberg Depression Rating Scale (MADRS).

How do we treat depression?

Two important reviews of psychopharmacology and CVD [5,6] demonstrate the safety, efficacy, and tolerance of antidepressants in patients with CVD.

Selective serotonin reuptake inhibitors (SSRIs) are the first-line treatment for depression in CAD patients. They include: fluoxetine, paroxetine, sertraline, fluvoxamine, citalopram, and escitalopram. SSRI are effective and safe. A recent study [7] focusing on escitalopram prescribed for 24 weeks in patients with depression following a recent acute coronary syndrome reported a lower incidence of MI in the escitalopram group than in the placebo group (8.7% versus 15.2%) after 8 years follow-up. A meta-analysis performed by Mazza et al. [8] showed that treatment with SSRIs results in significantly lower re-hospitalization rates in patients recovering from acute coronary syndrome (ACS) [8].

The antidepressant effects on the pathogenesis of CAD which might contribute to better clinical outcomes include:

a) anti-thrombotic: decreasing platelet activation (especially sertraline and paroxetine)

b) coagulation: reducing fibrinogen serum levels

c) sympathetic hyperactivity: decreasing sympathetic tone

d) inflammation: lowering hs-CRP, interleukin 6 (IL-6), and tumour necrosis factor-alpha (TNF-α) serum levels

e) insulin sensitivity and adiponectin levels: increasing levels of brain-derived neurotrophic factor (BDNF) and insulin-like growth factor 1 (IGF-1)

f) oxidative stress: reduction by changes on myeloperoxidase serum levels.

SSRIs have been shown to be safe because they do not slow cardiac conduction, do not cause orthostatic hypotension, and are well tolerated in terms of side effects. However, caution is necessary regarding pharmacological interactions. The most important pharmacological interactions of SSRIs in patients with CVD are those with anticoagulant therapy, as they increase the risk of gastrointestinal bleeding, and those with beta-blockers and anti-arrhythmic drugs related to QT prolongation. Another clinical context is heart failure with the potential for drug interactions between SSRIs and ACE inhibitors, angiotensin II receptor blockers (ARBs), beta-blockers, diuretics, and the valsartan/sacubitril angiotensin receptor-neprilysin inhibitor. In this case monitoring BP for possible hypotension is crucial. Care should be taken when prescribing ivabradine with citalopram, escitalopram, fluoxetine, venlafaxine, tricyclics, and trazodone, and QT interval monitoring is recommended [9]. Since SSRIs, with their higher serotonin affinity, are more likely to increase the risk of gastrointestinal bleeding, a proton-pump inhibitor should be added [10]. Fluvoxamine and fluoxetine increase warfarin serum levels via inhibitory effects on cytochrome P450 enzymes, in this case inhibition of CYP2C9, and should not be used with clopidogrel.

Other antidepressants which can be used with CVD patients are as follows.

• Serotonin norepinephrine reuptake inhibitors (SNRIs): the SNRI venlafaxine is a potent antidepressant which is dose dependent. In severe depression it can be titrated up to 300 mg/day. Venlafaxine may increase diastolic pressure, which is also dose dependent. It should be used in cases of moderate to severe major depression in cardiac patients if SSRIs fail.

- Noradrenergic and specific serotonergic antidepressants (NaSSAs) work by antagonism of both α_2-adrenergic and serotonin receptors. The NASSA mirtazapine has two important effects. First it can improve sleep, which is useful in cases of depressed patients with insomnia. Second, it increases appetite, which is of benefit for patients with anorexia. It also has a good response and tolerance in elderly patients.
- Norepinephrine–dopamine reuptake inhibitors (NDRIs): the NDRI bupropion is mostly in the context of smoking cessation.
- Melatonin receptor (MT1/MT2) agonist and serotonergic receptor 5HT2C antagonist agomelatine: used in the context of sleep disorder.
- Tricyclics (TCAs): norepinephrine–serotonin reuptake inhibitors and competitive antagonists of muscarinic, histaminergic, and α_1 and α_2 adrenergic receptors. The TCAs amitriptiline, clomipramine, and nortriptiline were the drugs of choice for depression in the 1980s. Although very effective, they were substituted by new antidepressants with fewer side effects (Box 12.1). TCAs are not recommended for treating depression in patients with CVD [11,12].

Clinicians should be very vigilant about potential adverse reactions, and ECG control during therapy may be suggested.

The following protocol should be used when prescribing antidepressants.

a) Start with low doses.
b) Titrate dosage slowly.
c) Always monitor closely.
d) Do not stop treatment immediately after achieving positive effects on psychological state of the patient.

Box 12.1 Side effects of TCAs

- Orthostatic hypotension—nortriptyline is the least likely to cause this.
- Slowing intraventricular conduction—increased QRS, PR, and QTc intervals on ECG. In overdose, it may lead to a complete heart block or ventricular re-entry arrhythmias.
- Tachycardia.
- Sedation is the most common side effect and is a result of anticholinergic and antihistaminic effects.
- Anticholinergic side effects—dry mouth, constipation, urinary retention, blurred vision, confusion, and delirium. Narrow-angle glaucoma can be aggravated.
- Sexual function side effects—frequent.
- A discontinuation syndrome related to cholinergic and serotonergic rebound. After prolonged treatment, TCAs should be tapered gradually over several weeks.
- Cardiotoxicity—overdose can be fatal.

Is treatment of depression in cardiac patients able to reduce mortality?

If clinical depression in patients with CAD increases the risk of cardiac events and mortality, it is reasonable to ask whether treatment of depression will reduce mortality and the risk of cardiac events. Until recently the answer was negative, based on a number of randomized trials:

Sertraline Anti-Depressant Heart Attack Trial (SADHAT) [13]

Sertraline Anti-Depressant Heart Attack Randomized Trial SADHART [14]

Myocardial Infarction and Depression—Intervention Trial (MIND-IT) [15]

Canadian Cardiac Randomized Evaluation of Antidepressant and Psychotherapy Efficacy Trial (CREATE) [16]

Enhancing Recovery in Coronary Heart Disease Study (ENRICHD) [17].

Most intervention trials of depression treatment conducted in cardiac patients were successful in treating symptoms and improving patient HRQol but failed to show a CV benefit, since they were not powered to detect a potential survival benefit. Therefore the question remains: Do patients with CAD who have been diagnosed with depression and referred to treatment have a better outcome than patients with untreated depressive symptoms?

In the ENRICHD trial [17] the effects of treating depression and low perceived social support on clinical events after MI were studied using cognitive behavioural therapy (CBT) as the standard intervention and sertraline as the drug of choice. The study failed to show a reduction in cardiac mortality, but this was due to distortion of the results by depressed patients who were resistant to treatment [18]. After exclusion of the non-responders, the analysis showed a reduced mortality in depressed post-MI patients treated with sertraline and CBT.

In the Translational Research Investigating Underlying Disparities in Acute Myocardial Infarction Patients' Health Status (TRIUMPH) registry 759 of 4062 patients with AMI met the criteria for depression, and 231 patients were treated compared with 528 untreated patients. When comparing the one-year mortality rates, post-MI patients with treated depression had a lower mortality rate than untreated depressed patients (6.7% versus 10.8%, adjusted hazard ratio 1.91, 95% confidence interval 1.39–2.62) [19].

These results require further replication in carefully designed randomized clinical trials to test whether depression screening and subsequent treatment are associated with better CV outcomes. Until then, as depression is an important comorbidity and treatment options are available but underused, it is reasonable to screen and treat depression independent of whether treatment benefits on CV outcomes exist [20].

Psychotherapy

In the ENRICHD trial [17], cognitive behavioural therapy was studied in combination with sertraline. The results showed that the intervention significantly decreased depressive symptoms but had no impact on all-cause mortality or AMI recurrence [17]. In 2018, the updated Cochrane Review [21] concluded that, for people with CAD, there was no evidence that psychological treatments had an effect on total mortality, the risk of revascularization procedures, or the rate of non-fatal AMI, although the rate of cardiac mortality was slightly reduced and psychological symptoms (depression, anxiety, or stress) were alleviated. Other psychological treatments such as interpersonal psychotherapy [16] and supportive stress management [22] have been tested, but shown small benefits.

The impact of psychological interventions on mortality is still a research field. No trial of psychological intervention alone has yet been associated with a reduction in CV outcomes or mortality. However, there is a consensus that CBT is effective in reducing depressive and anxiety symptoms among CV patients [23], and that, in some patients, a combined approach (psychotherapy and antidepressants) is better than either treatment alone in alleviating depressive symptoms and improving quality of life [24].

Conclusion

a) Clinical depression or depressive symptoms in patients with CAD increase the risk of fatal and non-fatal cardiac events and all-cause mortality.

b) Depression must be screened in CAD patients and treated.

c) SSRIs are the first-line antidepressants for treatment of depression in CAD patients.

d) Care should be taken with side effects and the interactions between antidepressants and medications used for treatment of CAD.

e) Cardiac patients on antidepressant treatment should always be monitored.

f) Antidepressants prescribing protocol: always start with low doses; titrate dose slowly and monitor closely; do not stop treatment too soon.

References

1. Williams ED, Steptoe A. The role of depression in the etiology of acute coronary syndrome. *Curr Psychiatry Rep* 2007; 9: 486–92.

2. Lichtman JH, Froelicher ES, Blumenthal JA, et al. Depression as a risk factor for poor prognosis among patients with acute coronary syndrome. Systematic review and recommendations: a scientific statement from the American Heart Association. *Circulation* 2014; 129: 1350–69.

3. American Psychiatric Association. Depressive disorders. In: *American Psychiatric Association: Diagnostic and Statistical Manual of Mental Disorders* (5th edn). Arlington, VA, American Psychiatric Association, 2013, pp 155–88.

4. Kroenke K, Spitzer RL, Williams JB. The Patient Health Questionnaire-2. Validity of a two-item depression screener. *Med Care* 2003; 41: 1284–92.

5. Chang L, Liu N. The safety, efficacy, and tolerability of pharmacological treatment of depression in patients with cardiovascular disease: a look at antidepressants and integrative approaches. *Heart Mind (Mumbai)* 2017; **1**: 8–16.

6. Piña IL, Di Palo KE, Ventura HO. Psychopharmacology and cardiovascular disease. *J Am Coll Cardiol* 2018; 71: 2346–59.

7. Kim JM, Stewart R, Lee YS, et al. Effect of escitalopram vs placebo treatment for depression on long-term cardiac outcomes in patients with acute coronary syndrome. *JAMA* 2018; 320: 350–8.

8. Mazza M, Lotrionte M, Biondi-Zoccai G, et al. Selective serotonin reuptake inhibitors provide significant lower re-hospitalization rates in patients recovering from acute coronary syndromes: evidence from a meta-analysis. *J Psychopharmacol* 2010; 24: 1785–92.

9. De La Cruz, Chionglo AM, Tran T. Current updates regarding antidepressant prescribing in cardiovascular dysfunction. *American College of Cardiology: Expert Analysis*, 7 January 2019. www.acc.org/latest-in-cardiology/articles/2019/01/04/07/59/current-updates-regarding-antidepressant-prescribing-in-cv-dysfunction.

10. Castro VM, Gallagher PJ, Clements CC, et al. Incident user cohort study of risk for gastrointestinal bleed and stroke in individuals with major depressive disorder treated with antidepressants. *BMJ Open* 2012; doi:10.1136/bmjopen-2011-000544.

11. Glassman AH, Preud'homme XA. Review of the cardiovascular effects of heterocyclic antidepressants. *J Clin Psychiatry* 1993; 54(Suppl): 16–22.

12. Pacher P, Kecskemeti V. Cardiovascular side effects of new antidepressants and antipsychotics: new drugs, old concerns? *Curr Pharm Des* 2004; 10: 2463–75.

13. Shapiro PA, Lespérance F, Frasure-Smith N, et al. An open-label preliminary trial of sertraline for treatment of major depression after acute myocardial infarction (the SADHAT Trial). Sertraline Anti-Depressant Heart Attack Trial. *Am Heart J* 1999; 137: 1100–6.

14. Glassman AH, O'Connor CM, Califf RM, et al. Sertraline treatment of major depression in patients with acute MI or unstable angina. *JAMA* 2002; 288: 701–9.

15. van den Brink RH, van Melle JP, Honig A, et al. Treatment of depression after myocardial infarction and the effects on cardiac prognosis and quality of life: rationale and outline of the Myocardial INfarction and Depression-Intervention Trial (MIND-IT). *Am Heart J* 2002; 144: 219–25.

16. Lespérance F, Frasure-Smith N, Koszycki D, et al. Effects of citalopram and interpersonal psychotherapy on depression in patients with coronary artery disease: The Canadian Cardiac Randomized Evaluation of Antidepressant and Psychotherapy Efficacy (CREATE) trial. *JAMA* 2007; 297: 367–79.

17. Berkman LF, Blumenthal J, Burg M, et al. Enhancing Recovery in Coronary Heart Disease Patients Investigators (ENRICHD). Effects of treating depression and low perceived social support on clinical events after myocardial infarction: the Enhancing Recovery in Coronary Heart Disease Patients (ENRICHD) randomized trial. *JAMA* 2003; 289: 3106–16.

18. Banankhah SK, Friedmann E, Thomas S. Effective treatment of depression improves post-myocardial infarction survival. *World J Cardiol* 2015; 7: 215–23.

19. Smolderen K, Buchanan D, Gosch K, et al. Depression treatment and 1-year mortality following acute myocardial infarction: insights from the TRIUMPH registry. *Circulation* 2017; 135: 1681–9.

20. Davidson K. 'Waiting for Godot'—engaging in discussions about depression care in patients with acute myocardial infarction while waiting for a definitive trial that never appears. *Circulation* 2017; 135: 1690–2.

21. Richards SH, Anderson L, Jenkinson CE, et al. Psychological interventions for coronary heart disease: Cochrane Systematic Review and meta-analysis. *Eur J Prev Cardiol* 2018; 25: 247–59.

22. Freedland KE, Skala JA, Carney RM, et al. Treatment of depression after coronary artery bypass surgery: a randomized controlled trial. *Arch Gen Psychiatry* 2009; 66: 387–96.

23. Reavell J, Hopkinson M, Clarkesmith D, Lane DA. Effectiveness of cognitive behavioral therapy for depression and anxiety in patients with cardiovascular disease: a systematic review and meta-analysis. *Psychosom Med* 2018; 80: 742–53.

24. Kronish IM, Krupka DJ, Davidson KW. How should we treat depression in patients with cardiovascular disease? *Dialog Cardiovasc Med* 2012; 17: 126–33.

Further reading

Freedland KE, Steinmeyer BC, Carney RM, et al. Use of the PROMIS® Depression scale and the Beck Depression Inventory in patients with heart failure. *Health Psychol* 2019; 38: 369–75.

Menke A. Is the HPA axis as target for depression outdated, or is there a new hope? *Front Psychiatry* 2019; 10: 101.

Song X, Song J, Shao M, et al. Depression predicts the risk of adverse events after percutaneous coronary intervention: a meta-analysis. *J Affect Disord* 2020; 266: 158–64.

Chapter 13

Management of non-conventional risk factors

Roberto Pedretti

Summary

Evidence supports the association of some non-conventional or yet to be established risk factors (RFs), such as serum uric acid (UA) or high-sensitivity C-reactive protein (hs-CRP), with the risk of arterial hypertension (HTN), metabolic syndrome, and chronic kidney disease and a worse prognosis in patients with known coronary vascular disease (CVD). However, there is no evidence from randomized controlled trials to support their use in guiding therapy. In the secondary prevention setting, detection of peripheral vascular damage and kidney dysfunction may provide significant additional prognostic implications.

111

Introduction

Preventive cardiology is a comprehensive multidisciplinary intervention aimed at the promotion of cardiovascular health in both primary and secondary prevention settings (which includes cardiac rehabilitation (CR)) [1].

Secondary prevention and CR programmes include comprehensive professional lifestyle interventions based on behavioural models of change (i.e. smoking cessation, healthy food choices, and exercise training (ET)) and conventional RF management [1]. The latter consists of effective control of blood pressure, lipids, and glucose in order to reach defined targets. The appropriate prescription of and adherence to cardioprotective drugs is an integral part of this approach [1]. Finally, psychosocial and vocational support are required to help patients to regain good health-related quality of life [1,2].

From time to time, new biological markers and certain clinical conditions which affect prognosis in patients with CVD are proposed as new RFs. Their role in clinical practice is discussed in this chapter.

Uric acid

Serum UA is not mentioned as a cardiovascular RF in the 2016 European Guidelines on CVD prevention [3]. Nevertheless, evidence supports the independent association of high serum UA levels with the risk of HTN, metabolic syndrome, chronic kidney disease, and CVDs [4]. A significant association with hyperuricaemia was found in patients with established coronary artery disease (CAD). In 13,273 patients with CAD, hyperuricaemia was found in 36.5% of men (>7.0 mg/dl) and 50.3% of women (>5.7 mg/dl). After adjustment using a multivariate Cox analysis, UA predicted one-year mortality with hazard ratios of 1.17 in men and 1.25 in women for each standard deviation increase in the natural logarithm [5]. In a follow-up of 1224 patients after acute myocardial infarction, increased serum UA was significantly associated with 30-day (odds ratio of the fourth quartile of serum UA concentration, 5.63) and long-term (adjusted odds ratio of the fourth quartile of serum UA, 3.72) all-cause mortality [6]. Serum UA is associated with increased risk of incident heart failure (HF), and with increased mortality risk in patients with existing systolic HF [7].

However, to date there is no evidence from randomized controlled trials that treatment of asymptomatic hyperuricaemia improves prognosis [4].

Circulating and urinary biomarkers

Biomarkers can be classified into inflammatory (e.g. hs-CRP), thrombotic (e.g. homocysteine, lipoprotein-associated phospholipase A2), glucose- and lipid-related (e.g. apolipoproteins), and organ-specific markers.

Hs-CRP is one of the most extensively studied and discussed biomarkers and consistently been shown to be a RF across large prospective studies. However, its contribution to the existing methods of CV risk assessment in secondary prevention is probably small [8], and the ultimate proof of risk reduction by selective anti-inflammatory treatment in a clinical trial has remained elusive for decades [9]. This may have changed with the results of the Canakinumab Anti-Inflammatory Thrombosis Outcomes Study (CANTOS), a randomized controlled double-blind trial involving high-risk patients with prior MI and a residual inflammatory status (defined by hs-CRP levels >2 mg/L despite intensive statin therapy) who were randomized to canakinumab (50, 150, or 300 mg every 3 months) or placebo [10]. Canakinumab, a human monoclonal antibody targeting interleukin-1β as the master cytokine of innate immunity, dose dependently reduced hs-CRP and interleukin-6 levels by ≤43% from baseline. At a dose of 150 mg (but not at the other doses), canakinumab significantly lowered the risk for the primary endpoints (MI, stroke, CV death) and secondary endpoints (hazard ratios, 0.85 and 0.83, respectively).

The vast majority of the other circulating and urinary biomarkers have no or only limited proven ability to improve risk classification, whereas organ-specific biomarkers may be useful for guiding therapy in specific circumstances.

Genetic markers

Genetic screening and counselling are effective in some conditions, such as familial hypercholesterolaemia [1]. Several genome-wide association studies have identified candidate genes associated with CVDs. Since the effect of each genetic polymorphism is small, most studies have used genetic scores to summarize the genetic component [1]. Given the lack of agreement regarding which genetic marker should be included, how genetic risk scores should be calculated, and uncertainties about improvement in CV risk prediction, the use of genetic markers in secondary prevention is not yet recommended in daily practice.

Epigenetics studies the chemical changes in the DNA that affect gene expression. Methylation of genes related to CV RFs is associated with variations in CV RF levels [11,12], and lower DNA methylation levels are associated with an increased risk of CAD and stroke [13]. However, there is no information regarding the effect of epigenetic markers in secondary prevention beyond conventional RFs. Thus epigenetic screening is not recommended.

Vascular damage

Routine screening with imaging modalities to predict future CV events is generally not recommended in primary prevention. They are considered as risk modifiers in individuals with CV RF scores around the decisional thresholds [1]. While coronary artery calcium score or arterial stiffness are not useful for prognostic stratification in secondary prevention, peripheral artery disease (PAD) is considered to be a very important marker of additional risk in patients with known CAD [14]. Therefore carotid ultrasound, measurement of the ankle–brachial index, and ultrasound study of the abdominal aorta and renal and inferior limb arteries may provide significant prognostic information.

PAD is associated with greater coronary atherosclerotic burden and progression in patients with CAD, regardless of its type, clinical setting, endpoints, or follow-up periods [14]. Moreover, in CAD patients there is a graded risk of death and non-fatal events as a function of the number of vascular beds affected. Secondary prevention strategies with intensive CV risk modification, antiplatelet therapies, and high-intensity statin treatment are needed, and are associated with an improvement in prognosis [14].

However, there is a gap in evidence as to whether routine screening for asymptomatic PAD is related to improved outcomes [14]. Future large-scale studies focusing on the role of screening for asymptomatic PAD in well-characterized cohorts, such as CAD patients, the elderly, or individuals at high CV risk, are warranted [14]. In addition, future studies should compare different screening methods and apply standardized definitions [14].

Kidney dysfunction

The care of patients with coexisting heart disease, in particular HF combined with kidney disease, is a major clinical challenge in both the acute and chronic settings. This challenge will become even more evident in the future with the increasing incidence of both disorders [15].

From a pathophysiological perspective, the heart and the kidneys share a number of linked pathways [15]. They include altered haemodynamics and fluid overload, leading to renal venous congestion, a profound imbalance with regard to hormonal and sympatho-adrenergic status, and mechanisms induced by malnutrition and cachexia. Furthermore, conventional CVD RFs are shared, including persistent chronic inflammation, anaemia, metabolic changes, and other factors that contribute to the acceleration of vascular aging.

Importantly, in the specific context of cardio-renal and reno-cardiac interactions, strong clinical evidence for appropriate treatment approaches is absent [15]. This is the result of a limited number of clinical trials specific to the cardio-renal syndrome and the use of different terminologies related to renal dysfunction in the cardiology and nephrology literature [15]. Moreover, the lack of evidence-based treatments underlines the importance of preventive and early diagnostic measures, and highlights the need for investigating the underlying mechanisms involved in the development of acute or chronic cardio-renal syndromes with a focus on treatments [15].

Until further data are available, patients with HF (or heart disease in general) and renal dysfunction should be treated early by multidisciplinary teams including specialists in cardiology and nephrology. This interdisciplinary approach demands bi-directional professional interactions between specialties and the formation of new collaborations.

Conclusion

Some factors, such as UA and hs-CRP, are associated with an increased risk of mortality and morbidity in patients with known atherosclerotic cardiovascular diseases. Nevertheless, clear evidence about their usefulness in therapeutic decisional flow is lacking. Clinical or instrumental evidence of peripheral arterial disease and kidney dysfunction are strong markers for worse prognosis in the secondary prevention setting.

References

1. Piepoli MF, Corrà U, Adamopoulos S, Benzer W, et al. Secondary prevention in the clinical management of patients with cardiovascular diseases. Core components, standards and outcome measures for referral and delivery. *Eur J Prev Cardiol* 2014; 21: 664–81.

2. Pedretti RFE, Fattirolli F, Griffo R, et al. Cardiac prevention and rehabilitation "3.0": from acute to chronic phase. Position Paper of the Italian Association for Cardiovascular Prevention and Rehabilitation (GICR-IACPR). *Monaldi Arch Chest Dis* 2018; 88: 1004.

3. Piepoli MF, Hoes AW, Agewall S, et al. 2016 European Guidelines on Cardiovascular Disease Prevention in Clinical Practice. *Eur Heart J* 2016; 37: 2315–81.

4. Borghi C, Agabiti Rosei E, Bardin T, et al. Serum uric acid and the risk of cardiovascular and renal disease. *J Hypertens* 2015; 33: 1729–41.

5. Ndrepepa G, Cassese S, Braun S, et al. A gender-specific analysis of association between hyperuricemia and cardiovascular events in patients with coronary artery disease. *Nutr Metab Cardiovasc Dis* 2013; 23: 1195–1201.

6. Kojima S, Sakamoto T, Ishihara M, et al. Prognostic usefulness of serum uric acid after acute myocardial infarction (The Japanese Acute Coronary Syndrome Study). *Am J Cardiol* 2005; 96: 489–95.

7. Wu AH, Gladden JD, Ahmed M, et al. Relation to serum uric acid to cardiovascular disease. *Int J Cardiol* 2016; 213: 4–7.

8. Kaptoge S, Di Angelantonio E, Pennells L, te al. C-reactive protein, fibrinogen, and cardiovascular risk prediction. *N Engl J Med* 2012; 367: 1310–20.

9. Weber C, von Hundelshausen P. CANTOS Trial validates the inflammatory pathogenesis of atherosclerosis setting the stage for a new chapter in therapeutic targeting. *Circ Res* 2017; 121: 1119–21.

10. Ridker PM, Everett BM, Thuren T, et al. Antiinflammatory therapy with canakinumab for atherosclerotic disease. *N Engl J Med* 2017; 377: 1119–31.

11. Guay SP, Brisson D, Lamarche B, et al. DNA methylation variations at CETP and LPL gene promoter loci: new molecular biomarkers associated with blood lipid profile variability. *Atherosclerosis* 2013; 228: 413–20.

12. Wang X, Falkner B, Zhu H, et al. A genome-wide methylation study on essential hypertension in young African American males. *PLoS One* 2013; 8: e53938.

13. Baccarelli A, Wright R, Bollati V, et al. Ischemic heart disease and stroke in relation to blood DNA methylation. *Epidemiology* 2010; 21: 819–28.

14. Manfrini O, Amaduzzi PL, Cenko E, Bugiardini R. Prognostic implications of peripheral artery disease in coronary arteruy disease. *Curr Opin Pharmacol* 2018; 39: 121–8.

15. Schefold JC, Filippatos G, Hasenfuss G, et al. Heart failure and kidney dysfunction: epidemiology, mechanisms and management. *Nat Rev Nephrol* 2016; 12: 610–23.

Chapter 14

How to improve adherence to medication and lifestyle measures

Ana Abreu and Miguel Mendes

Summary

Pharmacological and non-pharmacological adherence are essential for reducing cardiovascular (CV) mortality and morbidity; however, non-adherence is a major issue. Correct medication intake is complex, in particular for certain groups of patients. Modification of habits and changing to a healthier lifestyle may be even more difficult. Nevertheless, factors influencing non-adherence and adherence facilitators have been identified, and specific strategies to overcome multiple barriers to both types of adherence are available. In this context, adequate health education and communication are fundamental. Models and theories of change and adherence and theories of behavioural change are presented in this chapter. New technologies, such as digital health tools, which assist patients and health professionals to maintain therapeutic goals, may be helpful. Participation in cardiac rehabilitation (CR) and secondary prevention programmes with a multifaceted approach can also improve adherence.

Introduction

A World Health Organization (WHO) report states that the magnitude of non-adherence to medication and the scope of its sequelae are so alarming that more health benefits would result worldwide from improving adherence to existing medical treatments than from developing new ones. The WHO recognizes two distinct categories of non-adherence—preventable (patient forgets or misunderstands) and non-preventable (life-threatening side effects)—and recommends targeting tailored treatment interventions for the former [1].

Despite the recognition of pharmacological non-adherence as a major problem, this issue remains largely unsolved with a resultant high impact on mortality and morbidity [2,3]. Non-pharmacological non-adherence is not a minor problem, as habits are difficult to change. Lifestyle modifications, such as quitting smoking, eating only healthy food, starting or increasing physical activity (PA) and exercise, sleeping well, avoiding stress, and performing relaxing activities, are usually problematic to achieve and even more difficult to maintain long term.

Therefore the establishment of treatment monitoring and adherence reinforcement strategies for chronic CVD patients is warranted [4].

Factors influencing non-adherence, non-adherence risk groups, and facilitators of adherence

Many factors influencing non-adherence centred on the individual patient, disease, treatment, and health systems have been identified, including low education level or economic status, therapeutic complexity, poor practitioner–patient relationship, depression, and old age [5,6]. Barriers to good adherence to medication have been well identified by general practitioners (GPs) [7], including factors associated with patients, GPs, drugs, and healthcare systems (Box 14.1).

Studies of groups at risk of non-adherence are very heterogeneous. However, young and very old age, stress and anxiety, dementia and other cognitive disturbances, alcohol abuse, low socio-economic status, poor literacy, and lack of time for appointments can all be considered risk factors for pharmacological non-adherence.

Facilitators for better medication adherence, related to the patient, physician, medication, and healthcare system, have also been identified at GP appointments (Box 14.2).

Box 14.1 Barriers to medication

The patient
Poor health literacy.
Incapacity for self-management.
Substitution of prescribed drugs for self-administered drugs.
Inadequate drug dosage administration.
Fear of drug effects.
Mixture/change of drugs prescribed by different physicians, not reported.

The physician
Brief appointments.
Medication not completely reviewed in consultation.
Directive attitude of doctors.
Doctors not coaching self-management.
Poor communication between health professionals.

The medication
Polypharmacy.
Complex medication.
Long-term medication.
Adverse effects.

Education

Education and support for patients regarding the disease and its management.

Information for patients and caregivers regarding the purpose of the medication and potential side-effects.

Clear and easily available healthcare information for patients.

Active role of pharmacies in providing information about drugs.

Patient–doctor relation

Continuity of care with a good patient–doctor relation.

Medical treatment coaching.

Establishment of feasible targets involving the patient in treatment decisions.

Interprofessional support structure

Good organized interprofessional link around the patient.

Assessment of medication intake before, during, and/or after the exercise training sessions.

'Polypills'

Combined pills preferred to reduce the number of pills that need to be taken.

Adapted from Kvangstrom et al. [7].

How to measure adherence

Adherence is considered as (at least) 80% prescription accomplishment in a given period of time [8]. Health professionals frequently overestimate patients' adherence because of erroneous perception [9]. Measurement-guided medication management using validated adherence scales successfully improved adherence in non-adherent patients and may be implemented in clinical practice.

No gold-standard medication adherence scale exists. The Measure Adherence Questionnaire (MAQ) [10], the Morisky Medication Adherence Scale (MMAS) [11], the Adherence to Refills and Medication Scales (ARMS) [12], the Brief Medication Questionnaire (BMQ) [13], and the Self-Efficacy for Appropriate Medication Use Scale (SEAMS) [14] are some of the most user-friendly non-specific scales for assessing treatment adherence. MAQ, which is also known as the 4-item Morisky Medication Adherence Scale (MMAS-4), is the shortest scale, the easiest to score, and the most adaptable at the point of care and across populations. However, MAQ only identifies barriers to non-adherence and not self-efficacy. When compared with MMAS-8, MAQ has poorer psychometric properties, but it is a good tool for screening and is widely used. Both SEAMS, which is a 13-question scale, and BMQ, which has three main question headings with multiple sub-questions, assess barriers and self-efficacy, but scoring is difficult [15]. The Brief Illness Perception Questionnaire (BIPQ) [16] and the Beliefs about Medicines Questionnaire—Specific (BMQ-S) [17] are useful scales associate with adherence, as the perception of disease and beliefs about the medicines directly influence adherence.

Specific strategies for promoting pharmacological adherence

The characteristics and effects of intervention to improve medication adherence are varied. In a Cochrane Review in 2014 [18] only a minority of randomized controlled trials with the lowest risk of bias showed improvement in both adherence and clinical outcomes; however, no common interventions were present in these studies.

Strategies to improve adherence are aimed at different levels [19]:

a) Drug dosages
   (1) Start therapy with smaller doses, initially divided during the day to establish the appropriate dosage.
   (2) Use a simple scheme with preferred single administration of drugs to decrease the number of pills needed. Avoid dividing pills.
   (3) Adjust the dose carefully, taking into account age, renal and hepatic function, comorbidities, side effects, and drug interactions.

b) Information and tools
   (1) Present verbal and written information regarding medication effects, side-effects, and interactions, and instructions about when to contact the physician very clearly (once or several times if necessary).
   (2) Confirm that the patient has understood the main messages, by repeating it, including when and how to renew the prescription and how to contact the healthcare team in the case of side effects or an emergency.
   (3) Use special pillboxes and memory helpers.
   (4) Produce a clinical registry of all medication and information and share it with other health professionals such as nurses.

c) Drug brands

Always prescribe the same brand (even generics) for patient's recognition of box colour, pill colour, and format, thus decreasing the likelihood of possible error. Differences in bioequivalence may be problematic for CV patients who are older, poly-medicated, and have poor literacy levels or have renal or hepatic failure.

d) Safety and efficacy
   (1) Identify secondary effects and interactions, and ensure safety as a medical routine in all consultations.
   (2) At all appointments verify routinely that the patient is taking all the prescribed medication, with patients bringing the boxes and explaining doses and daily schedule of drug intake.
   (3) Reconcile your prescription with the prescriptions of other physicians.

e) Patient and family involvement
   (1) Meet the patient and family, and gain an understanding of their characteristics, such as culture, habits, literacy level, anxiety status, and age.

(2) Actively involve the patient in self-management and self-control.

(3) Involve family members living nearby to help in adherence.

(4) Empathetically discuss with the patient and family members all the barriers, suspension, or dosage change of each drug.

(5) Include patient and family members in programmes of therapeutic education with topics related to pharmacological treatment.

f) Chronic prescription of drugs

(1) Avoid chronic prescription of non-essential drugs, such as sedatives and non-steroidal anti-inflammatory drugs.

In summary, medications and their instructions for use may be complex. Teaching strategies that employ effective communication techniques between patients and providers, and among providers, may be the single most important intervention to reduce misinformation about medication and poor adherence related to low health literacy [20]. Empathy and time availability from health providers are vital strategies to use in ensuring treatment adherence. Negative strategies, such as directive attitudes, forcing a treatment on a patient who refuses or does not understand it, and using negative criticism regarding the patient's doubts and barriers will promote non-adherence [21].

Specific strategies for promoting non-pharmacological adherence

Non-pharmacological non-adherence might be more difficult to overcome than pharmacological non-adherence because of the difficulty that patients may have in changing fixed habits. However, a relationship between medication adherence and lifestyle modification has been observed [22]. Patients with poor medication adherence should be identified and included in motivational education programmes to promote lifestyle modifications (as well as medication adherence) [22].

The following specific strategies can be useful.

a) Focus on healthy lifestyle changes. For example, obesity, which is difficult to modify, needs a good weight management programme, stressing the importance of combining diet with regular exercise, a good sleep pattern, and relaxation with stress-reducing activities (for hormonal balance).

b) Establish a plan for changes and a specific start date agreed with the patient. The patient needs to be responsible, confident, empowered, and should understand the best time to start (as soon as possible). Emphasize the positive effects of specific strategies and stress the need for long-term changes.

c) Set realistic and achievable goals and choose the easiest risk factor to modify first. Unrealistic goals will only result in disappointment and frustration. If the goal is attained, it will encourage further achievements.

d) Adopt new habits gradually. Make one change at a time, not all together, and allow time for the change to be established.

e) Engage in daily structured activities, including exercise. As far as exercise becomes part of the daily routine, the easier it will be to do it, thus helping attainment of other goals.

f) Make healthy eating a daily activity. Eating doesn't have to be monotonous. There are plenty of healthy choices to explore and adapt. A grocery shopping list, excluding unhealthy foods, will help selection.

g) Ensure that the habits adopted can be maintained. Changes need to be comfortable, so that continuation throughout life is guaranteed. A balanced diet and enjoyable exercise need to be maintained for the long term.

h) Encourage support from family and friends. This is probably the most important recommendation for success.

i) Include support from specific expert consultations. For example, smoking cessation appointments are advised if the patients want to have this support.

Cardiac rehabilitation: secondary prevention programmes and adherence

Secondary prevention via CR programmes helps to promote both pharmacological and non-pharmacological adherence through a multidisciplinary team intervention, although adherence to these programmes is not optimal. In EUROASPIRE IV [23], 51% of CAD patients were advised to participate in a CR programme; 81% attended at least half of the sessions (41% of the study population). Older patients, women, and patients with lower socio-economic status, unstable angina, elective percutaneous coronary intervention, a previous history of coronary disease, heart failure (HF), arterial hypertension (HTN), or disglycaemia were less likely to be advised to follow a CR programme. People who smoked prior to the recruiting event were also less likely to participate. In a Swedish cohort study, smoking, a higher burden of comorbidities, and distance more than 16 km from the CR centre, among other factors, were associated with non-attendance at CR for patients after acute myocardial infarction [24].

Few HF patients, who could potentially benefit substantially from CR, are included in these programmes. The barriers in this case include older age, low socio-economic status, low education level, and lack of resources or transportation, expertise for referral, and capacity in the healthcare system. Important disease-specific barriers are severity of the symptoms, level of disability, impact of comorbidities, and difficulties in incorporating exercise in daily life [25].

Therefore all patients eligible for CR need to be motivated, understand the benefits and be available (especially active workers), and the programmes should be enjoyable and not located too far from home or work. Physicians need to believe in the benefits of CR and systematically refer all eligible patients. Geographical and socio-economic barriers, as well as the lack of referral by physicians, are the main obstacles to CR.

Organizational factors may facilitate adherence: for example, relaxation training, diet classes, group-based psychological counselling, medication counselling, and lifestyle modification support in the programme, the presence of the CR medical director for more than 15 minutes a week, assessment of patient satisfaction, and provision of adequate space and equipment [26].

Home-based CR programmes, including telemedicine technologies, can help to improve adherence, especially for some groups of patients (HF, elderly patients) [27].

Models and theories of change and adherence

A number of models and theories for motivating adherence have been proposed.

a) Self-determination theory [28]: understanding the factors of internal and external motivation for adherence in order to encourage it.

b) Integrative model of change [29]: modification of behaviour related to health in several stages, with progressive change.

c) Self-efficacy [30]: perceived self-efficacy is related to people's beliefs in their own capacities to control their own functioning and the events that affect their own lives.

d) Motivational interview [31]: direct patient-centred intervention to stimulate behavioural change, helping the patient to explore and resolve ambivalence.

e) Social learning theory [32]: characterization of extrinsic and intrinsic factors that act in human learning processes, considering that new behaviours may be acquired by observing and imitating others in a social context.

Techniques for behavioural change

Techniques for behavioural change can be defined as the active component of a specific irreducible, observational, and reproducible intervention, which has the potential to change the determinants of behaviour and target behaviours, depending on what it is intended to influence [33]. There are many techniques, which could be applied to promote PA, weight control, healthy diet, smoking cessation, stress management, and drug adherence [33]:

a) Feedback: provide feedback regarding accomplishment of the target behaviour.

b) Monitoring: self-monitoring a behaviour or asking someone else to monitor it.

c) Memos: alarms, sticky notes, telephone calls and messages, e-mails.

d) Personal trust: stress patients' personal capacities, focusing on previous success.

e) Behaviour demonstration: social comparison with others' performance.

f) Importance: reflection with the patient on the importance of behaviour change.

g) Decision balance: weigh the arguments of benefits and disadvantages regarding the change of behaviour and the maintenance of behaviour.

h) Purposes: definition of the purposes of change, using SMART principles— **S**pecific (personalized), **M**easurable (can be evaluated), **A**chievable (possible for the patient), **R**ealistic (applicable to the patient), and **T**emporal (evaluated at a specific time) [34].

i) Planning: detailed planning of actions to develop with respect to a specific target—what, where, how, with whom. Choose a simple and easy first step.

j) Rewards: reward the effort and attainment of purposes.

k) Anticipation plan: plan how to act in the case of an obstacle or unexpected event by anticipating and avoiding the risk of relapse.

l) Stress management: relaxation techniques, meditation, positive thinking.

m) Social support: identification of needs and sources of social support of different kinds.

New electronic technologies

Limited human resources, time availability, and economic restrictions may be partially overcome by new technologies. Better understanding of the link between behaviour and medication adherence could facilitate the development of programmes, tools, and approaches that improve adherence, thus leading to lower disease burden [35].

The association between medication adherence for chronic conditions and digital health activity tracking has been studied. Adopters of digital health activity trackers tend to be more adherent to HTN, DM, and dyslipidaemia drugs, and adherence increases with tracking frequency. This suggests that it may be worthwhile to examine new ways of further encouraging medication adherence through programmes that promote health tracking and leveraging insights derived from connected devices to improve health outcomes. A better understanding of how to use digital health tools to drive medication adherence and subsequently reduce the cost of managing chronic diseases is necessary [36].

With respect to mobile technology (mHealth) interventions for improving medication adherence, the feasibility of a phone-based medication reminder programme aimed at improving medication adherence in patients with CAD has been studied [37]. Although the improvement in medication adherence was not statistically significant in this study, it may have significant impact in the future. Smartphones with computer technologies can promote adherence and coaching [38]. Technology will increasingly be used and will probably help many individuals, but development of technology needs continued input from both patients and providers on how to incorporate these advances into clinical care [39].

Conclusion

Improving adherence requires a multifaceted approach, engaging principles of both precision medicine and population health [40]. Because of their multidisciplinary design, the close patient–physician relationship, and the patient-centred cardiologist–generalist link, CR programmes are an excellent strategy for promoting patients' pharmacological and non-pharmacological adherence. Adoption of new technologies could be a promising approach to overcoming the barriers preventing patients from attending CR programmes and facilitating the adoption of alternative CR models such as home-based programmes, and should be implemented.

References

1. Sabaté E. *Adherence to Long-term Therapies: Evidence for Action. WHO Adherence Meeting Report.* Geneva: World Health Organization, 2003.

2. Osterberg L, Blaschke T. Adherence to medication. *N Engl J Med* 2005; 353: 487–97.

3. McCarthy R. The price you pay for the drug not taken. *Bus Health* 1998; 16: 27–33.

4. Spertus JA, Kettelkamp R, Vance C, et al. Prevalence, predictors, and outcomes of premature discontinuation of thienopyridine therapy after drug-eluting stent placement results from the PREMIER registry. *Circulation* 2006; 113: 2803–9.

5. Kleinsinger F. The unmet challenge of medication nonadherence. *Perm J* 2018; 22: 18–33.

6. Kripalani S, Henderson LE, Jacobson TA, et al. Medication use among inner-city patients after hospital discharge: patient-reported barriers and solutions. *Mayo Clin Proc* .2008; 83: 529–35.

7. Kvangstrom K, Airaksinen M, Liira H. Barriers and facilitators to medication adherence: a qualitative study with general practitioners. *BMJ Open* 2018; 8: e015332. doi:10.1136/bmjopen-2016-015332.

8. Osterberg L, Blaschke T. Adherence to medication. *N Engl J Med.* 2005;353:487–497.

9. Murri R, Antinori A, Anmassari A, et al. Physician estimates of adherence and the patient–physician relationship as a setting to improve adherence to antiretroviral therapy. *J Acquir Immune Defic Syndr* 2002; 31(Suppl 3): S158–62.

10. Morisky DE, Green LW, Levine DM. Concurrent and predictive validity of a self-reported measure of medication adherence. *Med Care* 1986; 24: 67–74.

11. Tan X, Patel I, Chang J. Review of the four item Medication Measure Adherence Scale (MMAS-4) and eight item Medication Measure Adherence Scale (MMAS-8). *Innov Pharm* 2014; 5: 165.

12. Kripalani S, Risser J, Gatti ME, Jacobson TA. Development and evaluation of the Adherence to Refills and Medications Scale (ARMS) among low-literacy patients with chronic disease. *Value Health* 2009; 12: 118–23.

13. Svarstad BL, Chewning BA, Sleath BL, Claesson C. The Brief Medication Questionnaire: a tool for screening patient adherence and barriers to adherence. *Patient Educ Couns* 1999; 37: 113–24.

14. Risser J, Jacobson TA, Kripalani S. Development and psychometric evaluation of the Self-Efficacy for Appropriate Medication Use Scale (SEAMS) in low-literacy patients with chronic disease. *J Nurs Meas* 2007; 15: 203–19.

15. Lavsa SM, Holzworth A, Ansani NT. Selection of a validated scale for measuring medication adherence. *J Am Pharm Assoc (2003).* 2011; 51: 90–4.

16. Petriea KJ, Maina J, Weinman J. The Brief Illness Perception Questionnaire. *J Psychosomatic Res* 2006; 60; 31–7.

17. Horne R, Weinman J, Hankins M. The beliefs about medicines questionnaire: The development and evaluation of a new method for assessing the cognitive representation of medication. *Psychol Health* 1999; 14: 1–24.

18. Niewlaat R, Wilczynsky, Navarro T, et al. Intervention for enhancing medication adherence. *Cochrane Database Syst Rev* 2014; 11: CD000011.

19. Mota T. Outras terapêuticas e interações medicamentosas. In Abreu A, Aguiar C, Mendes M, Santa-Clara H (eds). *Manual de Reabilitação Cardíaca.* Lisbon: Sociedade Portuguesa de Cardiologia, 2013.

20. Schillinger D, Bindman A, Wang F, et al. Functional health literacy and the quality of physician–patient communication among diabetes patients. *Patient Educ Couns* 2004; 52: 315–23.

21. Brown MT, Bussel JK. Medication adherence: WHO cares? *Mayo Clin Proc* 2011; 94: 16–21.

22. Lee LM, Kim RB, Lee KJ, et al. Relationships among medication adherence, lifestyle modification, and health-related quality of life in patients with acute myocardial infarction: a cross-sectional study. *Health Qual Life Outcomes* 2018; 16: 100–8.

23. Kotseva K, Wood D, De Bacquer G, et al. Determinants of participation and risk factor control according to the attendance in cardiac rehabilitation programmes in coronary patients in Europe: EUROASPIRE survey IV. *Eur J Prev Cardiol* 2018; 25:1242–51.

24. Borg S, Oberg B, Lindolm D, et al. Factors associated with non-attendance at exercise-based cardiac rehabilitation. *BMC Sports Sci Med Rehabil* 2019; 26; 11:13. doi: 10.1186/s13102-019-0125-9.

25. Conraads VM, Deaton C, Piotrowicz E, et al. Adherence of heart failure patients to exercise: barriers and possible solutions: a position statement of the Study Group on Exercise Training in Heart Failure of the Heart Failure Association of the European Society of Cardiology. *Eur J Heart Fail* 2012; 14: 451–8.

26. Turk-Adawi K, Oldridge N, Tarima S et al. Cardiac rehabilitation patient and organizational factors: what keeps patients in programs? *J Am Heart Assoc* 2013; 2: e000418.

27. Rawstorn JC, Gant N, Direito A, et al. Telehealth exercise-based cardiac rehabilitation: a systematic review and meta-analysis. *Heart* 2016; 102: 1183–92.

28. Ng JY, Ntoumanis T, Thogersen-Ntoumani C, et al. Self-determination theory applied to health contexts: a meta-analysis. *Perspect Psychol Sci* 2012; 7: 325–40.

29. Proshaska J, DiClemente CC. Transtheoretical therapy: toward a more integrative model of change. *Psychotherapy: Theory Res Pract* 1982; 19: 276–88.

30. Bandura A. *Self-Efficacy: The Exercise of Control.* New York: Freeman, 2004.

31. Bennett G (1992) Miller WR, Rollnick S. (1991) *Motivational interviewing: Preparing people to change addictive behavior.* New York: Guilford Press, 1991. *J Community Appl Soc Psychol* 1992;2: 299–300. doi:10.1002/casp.2450020410

32. Bandura, A. *Social Learning Theory.* Englewood Cliffs, NJ: Prentice Hall, 1977.

33. Michie S, Johnston M. Behaviour change techniques. In: Gellman MD, Turner JR (eds). *Encyclopaedia of Behavioural Medicine.* New York: Springer, 2013.

34. Doran GT. There's a S.M.A.R.T. way to write management's goals and objectives. *Manag Rev* 1981; **70**: 35–6.

35. Quisel T, Foschini L, Zbikowski SM, et al. The association between medication adherence for chronic conditions and digital health activity tracking: retrospective analysis. *J Med Internet Res* 2019; 21: e11486.

36. Ni Z, Liu C, Wu B, et al. An mHealth intervention to improve medication adherence among patients with coronary heart disease in China: development of an intervention. *Int J Nurs Sci* 2018; 5: 322–30.

37. Baig MM, Gholam Hosseini H, Connolly MJ. Mobile healthcare applications:system design review, critical issues and challenges. *Australas Phys Eng Sci Med* 2015; 38: 23–38.

38. Bosworth HB, Granger BB, Mendys P, et al. Medication adherence: a call for action. *Am Heart J* 2011; 162: 412–24.

39. Zullig LL, Blalock DV, Dougherty S. The new landscape of medication adherence improvement: where population health science meets precision medicine. *Patient Prefer Adherence* 2018: 12; 1225–30.

40. Anderson L, Sharp GA, Norton RJ, et al. Home-based versus centre-based cardiac rehabilitation. *Cochrane Database Syst Rev* 2017; 6: CD007130.

Further reading

Bullard T, Ji M, Ruopeng N, et al. A systematic review and meta-analysis of adherence to physical activity interventions among three chronic conditions: cancer, cardiovascular disease, and diabetes. *BMC Public Health* 2019; 19: 636–47.

Rivera-Torres S, Fahey T, Rivera M. Adherence to exercise programs in older adults: informative report. *Gerontol Geriatr Med* 2019; 5: 1–10.

Treskes R, Velde E, Schoones J, Schalij M. Implementation of smart technology to improve medication adherence in patients with cardiovascular disease. Is it effective? *Expert Rev Med Devices* 2017; 15: 119–26.

Chapter 15

Cardiac rehabilitation for geriatric and frail patients

Carlo Vigorito and Ana Abreu

Summary

The progressive ageing of populations leads to a high burden of elderly patients with cardiac disease and is associated with comorbidities, cognitive/psychological deterioration, disability, social deprivation, and frailty. All these conditions complicate the clinical course of cardiac disease and worsen the outcome. Cardiac rehabilitation (CR), as a multidisciplinary intervention, improves mortality, morbidity, re-hospitalization, physical function, and health-related quality of life (HQoL) in adult patients after acute cardiac events. Older patients without clinical complexity can follow a CR programme slightly different from that for middle-aged patients, mainly based on aerobic training, with similar functional improvement. CR for elderly cardiac patients with comorbidities, sarcopenia, or frailty should be based mainly on strength exercise integrated with aerobic and balance training, but the most appropriate exercise programme has yet to be defined. Future studies should test whether interventions tailored to the presence and severity of frailty are effective in improving specific outcomes, with particular reference to functional capacity, physical function, quality of life, disability, frailty, hospitalization, and institutionalization.

Introduction

The number of elderly people in Europe will rise from 87.5 million in 2010 to 152.6 million in 2060 [1]. Elderly patients develop chronic disease more frequently, particularly cardiovascular disease (CVD) which is often accompanied by other comorbidities, cognitive/psychological deterioration, social deprivation, and frailty, all leading to disability and death [2]. These conditions shift the paradigm of care from a medication-based to a multicomprehensive approach, aiming not only to reduce morbidity and mortality, but also to improve HRQoL, disability, re-hospitalization, and institutionalization [3].

Cardiac rehabilitation in the elderly

CR is a multidisciplinary intervention which includes clinical evaluation and stabilization, secondary prevention, exercise training, counselling on risk factors (RFs), psychological evaluation, and follow up, with the intention of reducing all functional consequences of an acute cardiac event [4]. It is effective in reducing mortality, morbidity, re-hospitalization, and symptoms, while improving functional capacity and HRQoL [5]. Therefore it is recommended in the 2016 ESC Cardiovascular Prevention Guidelines as a Class IA intervention in patients with an acute coronary syndrome, revascularization, or heart failure (HF) [6]. However, the scientific evidence is mainly based on large scale meta-analyses, systematic reviews, or registries including mostly middle-aged patients, thus excluding very elderly patients with advanced comorbidity or disability [5,7].

In small observational studies selectively enrolling older patients with age-compatible preserved physical activity and functional capacity, CR improved exercise capacity, body composition, coronary RFs, psychological state and HRQoL [8,9]. Other larger registries which enrolled elderly patients participating in CR have also reported reduced mortality or hospitalization. Nevertheless, the retrospective or observational nature of these studies [10] may be associated with possible selection bias and hidden confounders.

The general approach to an elderly cardiac patient referred to CR can be schematically presented in Figure 15.1 [11]. The exercise programme should be preceded, particularly in patients over 75 years of age, by a multidimensional geriatric

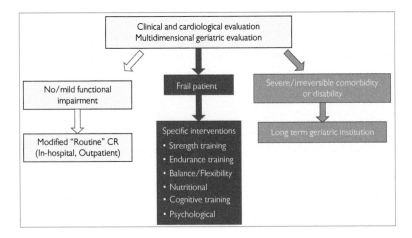

Figure 15.1 Approach to the elderly patient referred to cardiac rehabiliation.

Reproduced from Vigorito C, Incalzi RA, Acanfora D, et al. Recommendations for cardiovascular rehabilitation in the very elderly. *Monaldi Arch Chest Dis* 2003; 60: 25–39 with permission from Monaldi Archives.

evaluation (MGE) to exclude disability, cognitive problems, or frailty, conditions that require specific exercise protocols or approaches which are presented in more detail later in this chapter. If these conditions are excluded, the CR programme may have only small differences compared with that for young adult patients, and the intensity of the exercise programme should be tailored to the patient's functional state and prescribed according to peak heart rate (HR) achieved in a symptom-limited exercise stress test (EST) or to peak VO_2 achieved in cardiopulmonary exercise testing (CPET).

The training workload should initially be prescribed at a low to moderate intensity (50–70% of peak HR or 40–60% of peak VO_2). After 2–3 weeks of conditioning, the load can be increased, if tolerated, to a higher intensity level (70–85% of peak HR or 60–80% of peak VO_2) [12]. Peak exercise HR or peak Vo_2 are usually lower than in younger patients, because of age-related chronotropic incompetence, sedentary lifestyle, comorbidities, or drug side-effects (particularly beta-blockers). Therefore the training HR achieved at comparable percentage peak HR or peak Vo_2 is usually lower than in young adult patients, often close to that associated with light physical activity. What middle-aged patients consider as light exercise intensity (i.e. 2–4 METs) may be considered as moderate exercise intensity by elderly patients (<80 years) or even hard exercise intensity by very elderly patients (>80 years) [13]. If peak exercise HR cannot be used to determine the training workload (i.e. inability to perform EST, atrial fibrillation), the 20-point Borg Scale of Perceived Exertion (SPE) can be adopted, with a target of 11–13 for training intensity [14].

The frequency of sessions should range between three and four per week. In order to prevent exercise-induced symptoms or complications, exercise time and intensity should be gradually increased to achieve target HR and a session duration of 30 min. Programme duration may be similar to that of young adult patients (12 weeks), but elderly patients sometimes require additional weeks to reach optimal conditioning. Although treadmill training entails more skeletal muscle recruitment, elderly patients usually prefer training on a bicycle. However, the treadmill may be reserved for patients with good balance and physical function.

Resistance training (RT) on alternate days of aerobic sessions is recommended to counteract age-related loss of muscle mass, improve muscle strength and physical function, and decrease the risk of falls. These exercises can be performed with weight machines, dumbbells, or elastic bands at light to moderate intensity (60–70% of one repetition maximum (1-RM)) increased, if tolerated, to moderate to high intensity (70–85% 1-RM), with 8–12 repetitions involving six to eight groups of skeletal muscles. This set can be repeated two or three times, if tolerated, for a total duration of 40–60 min. A gradual increase in intensity, number of repetitions, and exercises is recommended, allowing 10 min rest between single exercises or a set of exercises. The Borg SPE can be used to evaluate the perceived strain of the patient, with scores of 11–12/20 and 13–14/20 corresponding to an intensity level between 60% and 80% 1-RM, respectively.

However, these programmes are unsuitable for very elderly patients with multiple comorbidities, physical functional limitations or disabilities, malnutrition, psycho-cognitive compromise, and frailty.

Frailty definition and evaluation

Frailty has been defined as increased vulnerability to stress characterized by declines in multiple physiological systems predisposing to a higher risk of negative outcomes, such as disability, institutionalization, and death [15]. The concept of frailty encompasses the physical, nutritional, cognitive, and psychosocial domains of health. Stemming from the two main models of frailty, the phenotypic model [16] and the accumulation of deficit model [17], several instruments have been used to evaluate frailty in very elderly patients in the community living population or in hospital settings [18].

Recently, frailty has been proposed for screening patients in the CV environment with poor prognosis. Depending on the diagnostic tool used, frailty has been described in 10–50% of elderly patients admitted for acute coronary syndrome/percutaneous transluminal coronary angioplasty (PTCA), trans-catheter aortic valve implantation, or HF [19]. In these studies, frailty proved to be an independent and powerful predictor of mortality, morbidity, and hospitalization. Currently, frailty evaluation for patients referred for CR is recommended for improving prognostic stratification and individualizing the rehabilitation protocol [20]. However, to date frailty has not been introduced as a standard method of assessment of very elderly CR patients, and it is still uncertain which diagnostic tool would be the best to be adopted in this setting. Different instruments, which are easy to use and able to assess many components of the patient's global health, could be utilized in clinical practice [18–20].

Sarcopenia, an important indicator of malnutrition, often overlaps with frailty, but it may also be present in very elderly patients who are not frail [21]. Sarcopenia is defined as a reduction of skeletal muscle mass and is evaluated by magnetic resonance imaging or computed tomography scanning (gold standard) or by the more practical DEXA scan or bioelectrical impedance analysis [22]. However, the majority of the tools for diagnosing frailty also include an evaluation of nutritional status, which provides an indirect clue to the presence of sarcopenia [18–20].

Cardiac rehabilitation in frail elderly patients

Multicomponent CR appears to be an ideal intervention for mitigating the high clinical risk burden of frail elderly patients after an acute cardiac event. Although frailty is present in a considerable proportion of elderly patients who are potential CR candidates [19], frail patients are poorly represented in CR studies because of selection bias and to logistical, economic, social, and cultural barriers. Therefore the true incidence and impact of frailty in CR is still unknown. Since frailty is increased in people over 75 years of age, all patients aged more than 75 referred to CR should have an MGE at admission, and have their training programme tailored according to the results of this evaluation (Figure 15.1) [11]. MGE requires a knowledge and utilization of specific evaluation tools, reflecting specific geriatric conditions with a strong impact on outcomes for elderly patients. Frailty scales used in elderly cardiology may be complex tools based on MGE [23] or derived from the phenotypic model [16] or the deficit accumulation model [17], with some modifications or adaptations. A recent call to action by the EAPC CR group recommended that CR cardiologists become familiar with these tools which have to be introduced in their routine patient assessment, particularly for patients aged over 75, possibly with the help of geriatricians [20]. Until standardization has been achieved, it is reasonable to adopt tools that have already been validated in the cardiology environment19. Recently, the Bern score, derived from the MGE, and the Essential Tool Subset (ETS) score (a very simple tool based on the haemoglobin level, the albumin serum level, cognitive impairment, and the chair rise test) have been utilized in patients undergoing transaortic valve implantation [24] and surgical aortic valve replacement, respectively [25]. Nevertheless, these and other instruments should be tested in CR patients.

Exercise interventions in frail patients

Exercise programmes for frail patients the should be tailored to the type and severity of their functional deficits and aim to improve global physical function, functional capacity, HRQoL, and neuropsychological status, to ensure safe transition of care, and to prevent re-hospitalization and institutionalization.

Many studies of frail patients living in the community, in hospital, or in a residential care setting have shown that multicomponent exercise protocols focusing particularly on resistance exercise, in addition to endurance, balance, and flexibility exercises, improve muscular strength, physical function, HRQoL, and balance, reduce the risk of falls, and preserve independence [26,27]. However, it is still uncertain how these exercise protocols can be transferred, with similar favourable results, to frail elderly patients enrolled in CR. Table 15.1 shows the RT protocol that can be adopted for sarcopenic or frail elderly patients aged over 75, as recommended by the EXPERT tool, a training and decision support system for optimizing exercise prescription in CVD [28]. Exercise intensity, the number of repetitions and sets, and the frequency of sessions should be gradually increased to reach the programme target, allowing sufficient time (5–10 min) between different types of exercises and sets. Clinical monitoring is also important for identifying symptoms, fatigue, or discomfort which should result in stopping the exercise and remodelling the whole programme.

Aerobic exercise training can be added on alternate days of resistance exercise, and should be prescribed according to baseline clinical and functional evaluation. However, in many frail patients with advanced physical limitations who are unable to perform a baseline EST or CPET, the aerobic training load (if the patient is able to stand on a bicycle or a treadmill) will be set at a heart rate slightly lower than that achieved in a 6 min walk test (6-MWT), starting with a session duration of 5–10 min and allowing a prolonged warm-up and recovery period. the Borg scale can be adopted to keep resistance or aerobic training intensity within safe limits, provided that the patients are able to report symptoms during exercise [14]. Heart rate, blood pressure, and clinical monitoring are helpful for minimizing the exercise-associated risk.

The intensity and frequency of strength exercises should be further reduced in extremely frail patients, with fewer skeletal muscles involved. Many of these patients

Table 15.1 Resistance training programme recommended for sarcopenic or frail elderly patients in cardiac rehabilitation

	Sarcopenia	Frailty
Type of exercise	Sufficient number of major muscle groups of upper and lower extremities (at least 6–8)	Reduced number of muscle groups involved, particularly lower extremities
Intensity levels	Moderate to high intensity 70–85% 1-RM	Low to moderate intensity 50–70% 1-RM
Number of repetitions per exercise	8–12	4–8
Number of sets	1–3	1–2
Frequency	2–3 per week	1–2 per week
Duration	40–60 min	Up to 40 min
Programme length	Up to 3 months	Up to 3 months

Reproduced from Vigorito C. Cardiac rehabilitation for elderly patients: possible and doable? In: New Opportunities in Cardiac Rehabilitation. *Medicographia* 2019;41:10-15. © Les Laboratoires Servier, France.

are not able to perform a 6-MWT, and may only require bed mobilization and postural training or supported walking [29].

High-intensity interval training (HIIT) may allow higher values of physical fitness to be attained in a shorter time in patients unable to tolerate a long aerobic training programme, but this exercise modality is not applicable to the majority of the frail elderly, as many of them are not able to tolerate very high exercise intensities.

There have been only a few reports of the results of exercise programmes in frail elderly patients admitted to CR. In very elderly patients after cardiac surgery, multicomponent interventions are tailored to the severity of frailty and improved physical function, balance, and HRQoL [29,30]. A multidisciplinary CR programme including individualized aerobic and resistance training improved functional capacity and HRQoL and reduced frailty in very old patients (>80 years) after transaortic valve implantation [24]. A tailored 12-week multicomponent exercise-based CR programme improved physical function and reduced re-hospitalizations in frail elderly patients hospitalized for acute decompensated HF [31]. Aerobic exercise combined with exercises for strength, flexibility, balance, and coordination significantly improved the Short Physical Performance Battery (SPPB) score in frail elderly patients after cardiac surgery [32].

Other components of cardiac rehabilitation interventions in elderly patients

Balance training is usually part of integrated exercise programmes, and includes static and dynamic balance components such as feet together, semi-tandem, tandem, and one-leg stand for 10–30 sec, side-stepping, and tandem walking. However, its effect on long-term independence and fall prevention is still uncertain [33]. Nutritional supplementation alone has a small effect on sarcopenia/frailty but, if combined with strength and endurance exercise, may contribute to reducing the severity of frailty [34].

Home-based CR, by improving patients' enrolment and adherence, is as effective as hospital-based CR [35], but the results in elderly and frail patients are still unclear. Tele-rehabilitation may improve cost-efficiency and delivery of CR in low- to moderate-risk cardiac patients [36]. However, it is uncertain whether modern technologies are applicable to high-risk frail elderly patients. In these environments safety is still an important unresolved issue.

Conclusion

Multicomponent CR is associated with favourable functional and clinical results, and should also be recommended for elderly patients. The modality and intensity of the prescribed exercise programme depends strongly on the baseline functional stratification and clinical status, which is identified using a multidimensional evaluation. In non-frail elderly patients aerobic training, adapted to age and integrated with RT, has positive effects on functional capacity, HRQoL, RF profile, and possibly mortality and re-hospitalization.

Frailty should be routinely assessed in CR patients, particularly those over 75 years of age, to increase prognostic power and guide exercise prescription. Standardization in evaluating frailty is needed, ideally a user-friendly instrument which combines ease of administration with the ability to reflect the major health domains of elderly patient. Preliminary data in frail patients admitted to CR programmes suggest that multicomponent exercise training, focused on RT, may improve functional capacity, muscular strength, mobility, balance, psychological state, and HRQoL, and reduce re-hospitalization. Further prospective studies enrolling adequate samples of frail elderly patients are needed in order to find the most effective and safest exercise training programme and hence improve specific outcomes in this frail population.

Case 1

An 82-year-old man with a non-STEMI and three-vessel disease treated with PTCA and a drug-eluting stent on the left anterior descending and right coronary artery (residual stenosis of 50% obtuse marginal artery) was transferred to CR 5 days after treatment. His clinical course was uneventful, but he reported some shortness of breath on light effort (NYHA III). Concomitant diseases were systolic hypertension, osteoarthritis, chronic obstructive pulmonary disease (COPD) stage II GOLD, and chronic gastritis with gastro-oesophageal reflux. He was a previous smoker of 10 cigarettes/day for 40 years, and was sedentary and slightly overweight. Echocardiography revealed a left-ventricular ejection fraction (LVEF) of 40%, left-ventricular (LV) hypertrophy, diastolic dysfunction pattern, and a borderline systolic pulmonary arterial pressure (PAP) of 35 mmHg. Medication included aspirin, clopidogrel, a beta-blocker, an ACE inhibitor, a proton pump inhibitor, a statin, and furosemide. Vital parameters on entry were: HR 68 bpm and blood pressure 132/86 mmHg. On a baseline symptom-limited ergometric stress test, the patient stopped at 4 min at a workload of 80 W and HR 124 bpm due to leg fatigue and shortness of breath, without any electrocardiographic evidence of myocardial ischaemia.

Frailty was assessed with an HB score (Table 15.2) derived from an MGE including the following items and scales: comorbidity (CIRS-G); nutrition (MNA), disability (BADL); physical performance and coordination (TUG); grip strength; gait speed by 6-MWT; cognitive status (MMSE); mood (GDS); functional capacity (6 min WT). This revealed CIRS 0.81, MNA 26, MMSE 24, GDS 10, TUG 15 sec, gait speed 0.68 m/sec, grip strength 21 kg, and no BADL deficit, resulting in a total score of 6 (no frailty).

The patient entered a supervised aerobic training programme on a bicycle, starting in hospital for the first three sessions and then continuing as an outpatient three times a week in combination with a home exercise programme. The aerobic training prescription was initially set at a low intensity (60% peak exercise HR, 76 bpm), and was cautiously increased to moderate intensity (75% peak exercise HR, 93 bpm) after 10 sessions. The session duration was 10 min for the first three sessions, and was gradually increased to 30 min.

RT sessions were added late in the morning, separated by aerobic sessions performed early in the morning. RT was preceded by measurement of a single-repetition

Table 15.2 Frailty based on MGE

Item	Quartiles	Score	Domain
MNA	≥25; 21–24; 17–20; <17	0–3	Nutrition
Katz activities of daily living (six activities)	0 = independence 1–2/6 deficit; 3–4/6 deficit; 5–6/6 deficit	0–3	Physical
Gait speed dividing 4.57 rn by time employed (rn/s)	≥0.9; 0.68–0.89; 0.58–0.67; ≤0.57	0–3	Mobility
Timed up and go (sec)	≤11; 12–19; 20–29; 230	0–3	Physical mobility and balance
Grip strength (kg)	Women: ≥15.7; 11.4–15.6; 7.3-11.3; ≤7.2 Men:≥30.6; 25.7–30.5; 19–25.6; ≤18.9	0-3	Muscular strength
MMSE	>24; 21–24; 16–21; ≤15	0–3	Cognition
Geriatric Depression Scale (15 questions)	<3; 3–5; 6–10; 11–15	0–3	Mood
Comorbidities (CIRS-G)	1 or 2; 3; 4; 5	0–3	Physical

Cutoffs: not frail, score 0–6; mild frailty, score 7–12; moderate frailty, score 13–18; severely frail, score 19–24.

maximal (1-RM) exercise. The RT intensity was initially set at 60–70% 1-RM, with gradual progression to 80% 1-RM and close supervision to prevent excessive straining. Exercises included leg extension, bench press, biceps curl, shoulder press, and leg press, with two sets of 8–12 repetitions for each exercise.

The home-based programme consisted of stair climbing two or three times a day and resistance exercises performed on non-hospital days using small dumbbells (0.5 kg).

After three months of training, the patient's grip strength had increased by 30% compared with baseline. When the bicycle exercise stress test was repeated the patient showed improved exercise tolerance (EST duration increased from 4 to 6 min, maximal intensity from 80 to 100 W, and peak HR to 130 bpm). Blood pressure was well controlled. He had some dyspnoea on exertion with moderate exercise (NYHA II), but he was able to perform all household and outdoor activities of daily life. He was able to walk 30 min, three or four times a week at a speed of 4–5 km/h.

Case 2

An 86-year-old female underwent transcatheter aortic valve implantation (TAVI) with a Medtronic Core Valve™ (Medtronic Inc., Minneapolis, MN, USA) for severe valve aortic stenosis. Associated comorbidities were hypertension, osteoporosis, osteoarthritis, COPD GOLD stage II, chronic kidney disease stage III (45 ml/min/1.73m²), previous colon adenocarcinoma treated with endoscopic resection, bilateral 50% carotid artery stenosis, and a previous transient ischaemic attack. She was very sedentary, reported fatigue and shortness of breath on minor effort, and limitations in housekeeping and outdoor daily living, requiring assistance for these activities. The patient had, a complicated clinical course post-TAVI characterized by anaemia requiring transfusion of two blood units, permanent pacemaker implantation, right femoral vascular haematoma, and moderate bilateral pleural effusion. Ten days after TAVI she was transferred to CR on ACE inhibitors, clopidogrel, proton pump inhibitors, and furosemide.

Her initial assessment during the in-hospital phase included clinical evaluation and transthoracic echocardiography. Baseline HR was 82 bpm and blood pressure 122/80 mmHg. Echocardiography showed LVEF of 55%, LV hypertrophy, diastolic dysfunction pattern, an enlarged left atrium, and mild systolic pulmonary hypertension (50 mmHg). She underwent MGE (Table 15.3). Her frailty score was assessed as indicated in Table 15.2 (moderate frailty).

The in-hospital rehabilitation programme included optimization of drug therapy, clinical control of peri-procedural complications, and nutritional intervention. Since the patient was unable to perform a functional test (6-MWT, EST, or CPET) for diagnostic and exercise evaluation tolerance purposes, a tailored programme was designed based on daily sitting calisthenics, assisted ambulation, RT of lower skeletal muscles at low load, and balance training. This programme took place in hospital for the first three weeks, and continued at home with in-hospital sessions twice a week. The home programme was designed with the assistance of a caregiver. It was based on lifting small weights (0.5 kg) 10 times for each arm, and stepping a few stairs twice daily.

Table 15.3 Frailty score

Item	Quartiles	Score	Domain
MNA	≥25; 21-24; 17-20; <17	0-3	Nutrition
Katz activities of daily living (six activities)	0 = independence 1-2/6 deficit; 3-4/6 deficit; 5-6/6 deficit	0–3	Physical
Gait speed dividing 4.57 m by time employed (m/s)	≥0.9; 0.68–0.89; 0.58–0.67; ≤0.57	0–3	Mobility
Timed up and go (sec)	≤11; 12–19; 20–29; ≥30	0–3	Physical mobility and balance
Grip strength (kg)	Women: ≥15.7; 11.4–15.6; 7.3–11.3; ≤7.2 Men: ≥30.6; 25.7–30.5; 19–25.6; ≤18.9	0–3	Muscular strength
MMSE	>24; 21–24; 16–21; ≤15	0–3	Cognition
Geriatric Depression Scale (15 questions)	<3; 3–5; 6–10; 11–15	0–3	Mood
Comorbidities (CIRS-G)	1 or 2; 3; 4; 5	0-3	Physical

Cut-offs: not frail, score 0–6; mild frailty, score 7–12; moderate frailty, score 13–18; severely frail, score 19–24.

After 12 weeks of CR, the geriatric evaluation was repeated. The results obtained are presented in Table 15.3. The patient was discharged home with good functional results; she recovered two abilities of daily living, improved her mobility, balance, and functional capacity, and slightly reduced her frailty status.

References

1. Directorate-General for Research and Innovation (European Commission). *Population Ageing in Europe: Facts, Implications and Policies*. Brussels: Publication Ofiice of the European Union, 2014.
2. Myers V, Drory Y, Gerber Y. Clinical relevance of frailty trajectory post myocardial infarction. *Eur J Prev Cardiol* 2014; 21: 758–66.
3. Rich MW, Chyun DA, Skolnick AH, et al. Knowledge gaps in cardiovascular care of the older adult population: a scientific statement from the American Heart Association, American College of Cardiology, and American Geriatrics Society. *J Am Coll Cardiol* 2016; 67: 2419–40.
4. Leon AS, Franklin BA, Costa F, et al. Cardiac rehabilitation and secondary prevention of coronary heart disease. An American Heart Association Scientific Statement from the Council on Clinical Cardiology (Subcommittee on Exercise, Cardiac Rehabilitation, and Prevention) and the Council on Nutrition, Physical Activity, and Metabolism (Subcommittee on Physical Activity), in collaboration with the American Association of Cardiovascular and Pulmonary Rehabilitation. *Circulation* 2005; 111: 369–76.
5. Anderson L, Oldridge N, Thompson DR, et al. Exercise-based cardiac rehabilitation for coronary heart disease. Cochrane systematic review and meta-analysis. *J Am Coll Cardiol* 2016; 67: 1–12.

6. Sixth Joint Task Force of the European Society of Cardiology and Other Societies on Cardiovascular Disease Prevention in Clinical Practice. 2016 European Guidelines on cardiovascular disease prevention in clinical practice. *Eur Heart J* 2016; 37: 2315–81.

7. Rauch B, Davos CH, Doherty P, et al. The prognostic effect of cardiac rehabilitation in the era of acute revascularization and statin therapy: a systematic review and meta-analysis of randomized and non-randomized studies—the Cardiac Rehabilitation Outcome Study (CROS). *Eur J Prev Cardiol.* 201; 23: 1914–39.

8. Marchionni N, Fattirolli F, Fumagalli S, et al. Improved exercise tolerance and quality of life with cardiac rehabilitation of older patients after myocardial infarction: results of a randomized, controlled trial. *Circulation* 2003; 107: 2201–6.

9. Menezes AR, Lavie CJ, Forman DE. Cardiac rehabilitation in the elderly. *Prog Cardiovasc Dis* 2014; 57: 152–9.

10. Suaya JA, Stason WB, Ades PA, et al. Cardiac rehabilitation and survival in older coronary patients. *J Am Coll Cardiol* 2009; 54: 25–33.

11. Vigorito C, Incalzi RA, Acanfora D, et al. [Recommendations for cardiovascular rehabilitation in the very elderly]. *Monaldi Arch Chest Dis* 2003; 60: 25–39 (in Italian).

12. Vanhees L, Geladas N, Hansen D, et al. Importance of characteristics and modalities of physical activity and exercise in the management of cardiovascular health in individuals with cardiovascular risk factors: recommendations from the EACPR (Part II). *Eur J Prev Cardiol* 2012; 19:1005–33.

13. Fletcher GF, Balady GJ, Amsterdam EA, et al. Exercise standards for testing and training. A statement for healthcare professionals from the American Heart Association. *Circulation* 2001; 104: 1694–1740.

14. Borg GA. Psychophysical bases of perceived exertion. *Med Sci Sports Exerc* 1982; 14: 377–81.

15. Clegg A, Young J, Iliff S, et al. Frailty in elderly people. *Lancet* 2013; 381: 752–62.

16. Fried LP, Tangen CM, Walston J, et al. Frailty in older adults: evidence for a phenotype. *J Gerontol A Biol Sci Med Sci* 2001; 56: M146–56.

17. Rockwood K, Mitnitski A. Frailty in relation to the accumulation of deficits. *J Gerontol A Biol Sci Med Sci* 2007; 62: 722–7.

18. Theou O, Thomas D, Brothers TD, et al. Operationalization of frailty using eight commonly used scales and comparison of their ability to predict all-cause mortality. *J Am Geriatr Soc* 2013; 61:1537–51.

19. Afilalo J, Alexander KP, Mack MJ, et al. Frailty assessment in the cardiovascular care of older adults. *J Am Coll Cardiol* 2014; 63: 747–62.

20. Vigorito C, Abreu A, Ambrosetti M, et al. Frailty and cardiac rehabilitation: a call to action from the EAPC Cardiac Rehabilitation Section. *Eur J Prev Cardiol* 2017; 24: 577–90.

21. Cruz-Jentoft AJ, Kiesswetter E, Drey M, Sieber CC. Nutrition, frailty, and sarcopenia. *Aging Clin Exp Res* 2017: 29: 43–8.

22. Cruz-Jentoft AJ, Bahat G, Bauer J, et al. Sarcopenia: revised European consensus on definition and diagnosis. *Age Ageing.* 2019; 48: 16–31.

23. Schoenenberger AW, Stortecky S, Neumann S. et al. Predictors of functional decline in elderly patients undergoing transcatheter aortic valve implantation (TAVI). *Eur Heart J* 2013; 34, 684–92.

24. Eichler S, Salzwedel A, Reibis R, et al. Multicomponent cardiac rehabilitation in patients after transcatheter aortic valve implantation: predictors of functional and psycho-cognitive recovery. *Eur J Prev Cardiol* 2017; 24: 257–64.

25. Afilalo J, Lauck S, Kim DH, et al. Frailty in older adults undergoing aortic valve replacement. The FRAILTY-AVR Study. *J Am Coll Cardiol* 2017; 70: 689–700.

26. Theou O, Stathokostas L, Roland KP, et al. The effectiveness of exercise interventions for the management of frailty: a systematic review. *J Aging Res* 2011: 569194.

27. de Labra C, Guimaraes Pinheiro C, Maseda A, et al. Effects of physical exercise interventions in frail older adults: a systematic review of randomized controlled trials. *BMC Geriatr* 2015; 15: 154–70.

28. Hansen D, Dendale P, Coninx K, et al. The European Association of Preventive Cardiology Exercise Prescription in Everyday Practice and Rehabilitative Training (EXPERT) tool: a digital training and decision support system for optimized exercise prescription in cardiovascular disease. Concept, definitions and construction methodology. *Eur J Prev Cardiol* 2017; 24: 1017–31.

29. Opasich C, Patrignani A, Mazza A, et al. An elderly-centered, personalized, physiotherapy program early after cardiac surgery. *Eur J Cardiovasc Prev Rehabil* 2010; 17: 582–7.

30. Busch JC, Lillou D, Wittig G, et al. Resistance and balance training improves functional capacity in very old participants attending cardiac rehabilitation after coronary bypass surgery. *J Am Geriatr Soc* 2012; 60: 2270–6.

31. Reeves GR, Whellan DJ, O'Connor CM, et al. A novel rehabilitation intervention for older patients with acute decompensated heart failure. The REHAB-HF Pilot Study. *J Am Coll Cardiol Heart Fail* 2017; 5: 359–66.

32. Molino-Lova R, Pasquini G, Vannetti F, et al. Effects of a structured physical activity intervention on measures of physical performance in frail elderly patients after cardiac rehabilitation: a pilot study with 1-year follow-up. *Intern Emerg Med* 2013; 8: 581–9.

33. Cadore EL, Rodrıguez-Manas L, Sinclair A, Izquierdo M. Effects of different exercise interventions on risk of falls, gait ability, and balance in physically frail older adults: a systematic review. *Rejuvenation Res* 2013; 16: 105–14.

34. Tze Pin Ng, Feng L, Nyunt MSZ, et al. Nutritional, physical, cognitive, and combination interventions and frailty reversal among older adults: a randomized controlled trial. *Am J Med* 2015; 128: 1225–36.

35. Anderson L, Sharp GA, Norton RJ, et al. Home-based versus centre-based cardiac rehabilitation. *Cochrane Database Syst Rev.* 20170; 6: CD007130.

36. Brouwers RW, Kraal JJ, Traa SC, et al. Effects of cardiac tele-rehabilitation in patients with coronary artery disease using a personalized patient-centered web application: protocol for the SmartCare-CAD randomized controlled trial. *BMC Cardiovasc Disord* 2017; 17: 46.

Further reading

Hoogendijk E, Afilalo J, Ensrud K, et al. Frailty: implications for clinical practice and public health. *Lancet*, 394(10206): 1365–75.

Dent E, Martin F, Bergman H, Woo J, et al. Management of frailty: opportunities, challenges, and future directions. *Lancet*, 394(10206): 1376–86.

Chapter 16

Return to work

Rona Reibis and Heinz Völler

Summary

The vocational reintegration of patients after an acute cardiac event is a crucial step towards complete convalescence from both the social and individual point of view. Residual job ability (partial, total/temporary, or permanent disability) depends on existing cardiac, psycho-cognitive and professional barriers. Return to work (RTW) rates are determined by left ventricular function, residual ischaemia, and heart rhythm stability, as well as by the occupational requirement profile, such as blue- or white-collar work, night shifts, and the ability to commute. Psychosocial factors, including depression, self-perceived health situation, and pre-existing cognitive impairment, determine the reintegration rate to a significant extent. Patients at risk of poor vocational outcomes should be identified early in the rehabilitation process in order to avoid failure of reintegration and to prevent social and professional exclusion with adverse psychological and financial consequences.

139

Introduction

Cardiac events increase the risk of poorer work conditions, including reduced spectrum of responsibility, part-time employment, lower salary, and premature dismissal. Irrespective of the initial treatment strategy, RTW rates within 12 months after acute coronary syndrome (ACS) vary from 67% to 93%. The mean time delay until RTW is two to three months. While the medical evaluation of the patient's ability to RTW is largely based on objective data such as cardiac function, including left ventricular ejection fraction (LVEF) and exercise capacity, as well as existing comorbidities, the patient's self-assessment mainly includes work-related factors (satisfaction with the previous work situation, negative expectations upon resuming work) and general well-being.

Predictors of return to work

Cardiac-related factors

LVEF at admission has been described as one of the most important prognostic clinical parameters for RTW. The patient's maximal endurance bicycle exercise capacity can be interpreted as an absolute value, as well as relative to body weight (Table 16.1). If there is a discrepancy between LVEF and exercise capacity, cardiopulmonary exercise testing may be performed to correlate peak VO_2 and metabolic equivalent (MET) achieved with the required professional performance. Imaging using pharmacological or dynamic stress echocardiography is not usually necessary for assessment of occupational reintegration. Exclusion of haemodynamically relevant cardiac arrhythmias is essential, particularly for occupational activities in which short-term arrhythmia-associated consciousness disorders may lead to potentially dangerous situations (professional drivers, roofers). Existing comorbidities (diabetes mellitus, renal failure, previous stroke, chronic obstructive pulmonary disease, peripheral artery disease (PAD)) also influence the RTW rate.

Psychosocial factors

Self-assessment of the patient's ability to perform the previous activity adequately has a high predictive value for reintegration. Professional reintegration is often limited by the fear of harming oneself because of work-related physical or emotional stress due to occupational physical and mental stress. Clinically detectable depression and anxiety disorders are significantly correlated with the absence of RTW. Thus the use of standardized psychometric questionnaires may be helpful. Frequent shift work, night work, or overtime may aggravate occupational stress. The barriers limiting RTW can be identified by involving professional groups within the scope of multidisciplinary rehabilitation [1], and correlating this with an assessment of the possibility for vocational reintegration (Figure 16.1).

Table 16.1 Estimate of maximum cardiopulmonary capacity and full-time working capacity on the basis of the achieved peak Vo_2 (German recommendations)*

Maximum capacity on the ergometer	Maximum capacity in relation to BW	Endurance capacity on the ergometer	Estimated energy expenditure (METs)	Work intensity
<50 watts	About 1 watt/kg BW	Up to 50 watts	<3.1	Very light
>50–75 watts	>1–1.5 watts/kg BW	>50–75 watts	<4.3	Light
>75–125 watts	>1.5–2 watts/kg BW	<75–100 watts	<6.4	Moderate
125–150 watts	> 2 watts/kg BW	>100 watts	<7.4	Heavy

*Example for a patient with a body weight of 80 kg.
BW, body weight; MET, metabolic equivalent.

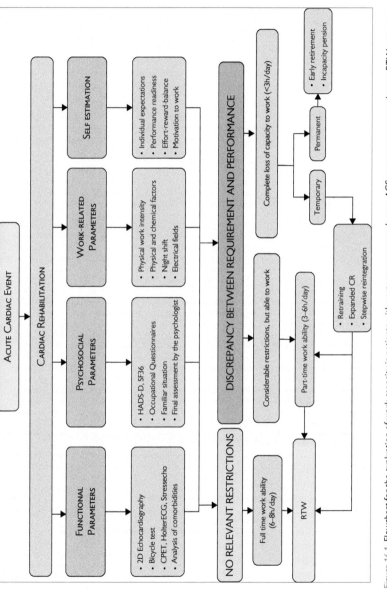

Figure 16.1 Flowchart for the evaluation of work capacity in patients with acute coronary syndrome: ACS, acute coronary syndrome; RTW, return to work; CPET, cardiopulmonary exercise testing; CR, cardiac rehabilitation; HADS-D, Hospital Anxiety and Depression Scale; SF-36, Short Form Health Survey 36.

Work-related factors

Working prior to a coronary event is highly predictive for RTW. Nevertheless the characteristics of the tasks performed are important for RTW probability. Work-related factors include the intensity of physical effort required as well as specific workplace conditions of a physical and chemical nature (toxic fumes, high pressure or low atmospheric pressure, high noise level, fine dust load, heat/cold, electric fields) which have to be considered. Psychological tasks including production line work, piecework, or working under time pressure are important professional parameters in the assessment of reintegration ability. The ability to commute (reach the workplace by walking, driving, cycling, or public transport) can be a limiting factor for patients with a driving ban. The occupational reintegration of patients with implanted electrical devices (cardiac pacemakers, defibrillators) may be difficult, especially in some industries. Given the possibility of electromagnetic interference with implanted electrical devices, this might constitute a contraindication for the resumption of work in certain jobs.

Practical guidance on reintegration strategies

Reintegration of patients after ACS should be considered as a multicomponent process including initial CR, after-care programmes, and expanded socio-medical support [2]. A practical model for adaptation to work after ACS should integrate human and work-related parameters for final RTW clearance.

Cardiac rehabilitation and return to work

Occupational recovery and subsequent professional reintegration can be significantly improved by CR. If a delay in fitness to work is predictable, various expanded reintegration strategies including prolonged rehabilitation, stepwise integration, or retraining have to be considered (Box 16.1). Rehabilitation programmes using novel digital technologies (web-based remote programmes) may be helpful, particularly for patients with a high professional performance [3]. As this eHealth-based form of

---

Box 16.1 Supportive strategies for professional reintegration during CR

- Risk stratification (identification of negative chronic occupational conditions).
- Work-related diagnosis (recording current job characteristics).
- Multiprofessional team meetings (cardiologists, occupational physician, social worker, physiotherapist, psychologist).
- Involvement of family members.
- Individual re-entry training (ergonomic interventions).
- Psychosocial counselling.
- Contacting the employer, discussion of reintegration strategy.
- Contacting pension insurance, if necessary.
- Organization of financial security.
- Exact recommendations in the case of reintegration failure.

CR is supervised remotely, patients are able to restart working while concurrently engaging in ongoing tele-CR.

Correlation of physical performance and work severity

RTW may be permitted if the patient's individual functional capacity is at least twice the energy demands of the specific work activity. The 2011 Compendium of Physical Activities [4], which correlates specific activities and measured or estimated MET values, can be used for individual job characterization. Workload frequently varies during the day so, in cases of uncertainty, the requirement can be assessed directly at the workplace. A controlled field study can analyse the objective CV demands by registering heart rate (HR) and VO_2 during several work tasks using portable oxygen uptake and HR monitors.

Driving ability in cardiac patients

The driving ability of cardiac patients is primarily dependent on their haemodynamic stability, the duration of the arrhythmia-free interval, and the type of driving licence they have [5]. In general, a distinction is made between private (cars and motor-cycles, group 1) and professional drivers (truck/lorry driver, bus driver, pilot, taxi driver group 2). A comprehensive UK fitness to drive recommendation, covering multiple CVDs, has recently been published [6].

References

143

Conclusion

In addition to medical factors, the reintegration of cardiac patients is primarily determined by psychocognitive and work-related parameters. RTW requires an increased effort and should preferably start without delay after completion of the post-event rehabilitation programme. Interdisciplinary support (cardiologists, psychologists, occupational physicians, general practitioners) is required, particularly for patients with at increased risk of reintegration failure.

References

1. Lamberti M, Ratti G, Gerardi D, et al. Work-related outcome after acute coronary syndrome: implications of complex cardiac rehabilitation in occupational medicine. *Int J Occup Med Environ Health* 2016; 29: 649–57.

2. Reibis R, Salzwedel A, Abreu A, et al. The importance of return to work: how to achieve optimal reintegration in ACS patients. *Eur J Prev Cardiol* 2019; 10: 1358–69.

3. O'Brien L, Wallace S, Romero L. Effect of psychosocial and vocational interventions on return-to-work rates post-acute myocardial infarction: a systematic review. *J Cardiopulm Rehabil Prev* 2018; 38: 215–23.

4. Ainsworth BE, Haskell WL, Herrmann SD, et al. 2011 Compendium of Physical Activities: a second update of codes and MET values. *Med Sci Sports Exerc* 2011; 43: 1575–81.

5. Vijgen J, Botto G, Camm J, et al. Consensus statement of the European Heart Rhythm Association: updated recommendations for driving by patients with implantable cardioverter defibrillators. *Eur J Cardiovasc Nurs* 2010; 9: 3–14.

6. Valentine C. Driving after an acute coronary syndrome. *BMJ* 2015; 351: h5988.

Further reading

Bresseleers J, De Sutter J. Return to work after acute coronary syndrome: time for action. *Eur J Prev Cardiol* 2019; 26:1355–7.

Salzwedel A, Wegscheider K, Schulz-Behrendt C, et al. No impact of an extensive social intervention program on return to work and quality of life after acute cardiac event: a cluster-randomized trial in patients with negative occupational prognosis. *Int Arch Occup Environ Health* 2019; 92: 1109–20.

Tiikkaja M, Aro AL, Alanko T, et al. Electromagnetic interference with cardiac pacemakers and implantable cardioverter–defibrillators from low-frequency electromagnetic fields in vivo. *Europace* 2013; 15: 388–394.

Chapter 17

Specific issues with physical activity after cardiac rehabilitation

Marco Ambrosetti and Esteban Garcia-Porrero

Summary

The transition between phase II (structured, supervised) and phase III (long-term, unsupervised) cardiac rehabilitation (CR) provides an opportunity to promote regular physical activity (PA) in cardiac patients, with the aim of maintaining functional capacity and improving cardiovascular (CV) prognosis. Unfortunately, barriers at the individual and organizational/environmental level may lead to poor adherence to PA, with a consequent need for a call to action by the whole multidisciplinary CR staff. In particular, improvement of patients' self-efficacy—defined as beliefs about one's ability to perform a specific action—is clearly associated with better adherence to the programme. The gold standard is individualized prescription of a PA plan—type, intensity, duration, and frequency—which should be monitored and revised periodically on the basis of serial direct evaluations of cardiorespiratory fitness. If this is not available, good PA practice focusing on training intensity and volume should be recommended. In selected cases, the delivery of a long-term PA programme could be supported by digital health tools.

145

Introduction

CR has evolved from exercise only into a comprehensive programme which also addresses CVD risk factors (RFs) and provides education and psychosocial support. Classically, it consists of three phases. Phase I refers to inpatient rehabilitation during the index hospitalization. Phase II refers to physician-supervised inpatient or (mostly) outpatient programmes for up to 4–6 months after the index event. Finally, phase III is usually an intentional exercise performed at home or another location remote from the monitored CR setting in the context of primary care.

The transition between phase II and phase III CR can be a vulnerable period: the termination of structured rehabilitation, whatever the outcome, generally leaves patients at increased risk of non-adherence to pharmacological therapies and lifestyle interventions. As a consequence, clinical stabilization may deteriorate, in that global

CV risk and functional disabilities may increase and thus attenuate, or even nullify, the positive effects of the rehabilitation programme.

Exercise training [1], defined as planned structured PA performed on a repeated basis over an extended period of time with the specific objective of improving cardiorespiratory fitness and global health, is the CR core component that patients most commonly fail to maintain. Activity maintenance rates currently exceed 80% in the first three months after initiation, but often fall to 20–30% a year after graduation from phase II CR. For these reasons, the maintenance of good PA in the long term is a cornerstone of CV prevention [2].

How to promote regular physical activity after phase II cardiac rehabilitation

Several barriers contribute to poor attendance at structured long-term PA (Table 17.1). Hence there is a need for CR staff to carry out systematic evaluation and action during the transition phase.

Research addressing adherence to PA during phase III CR has revealed that engaging in one-to-one exercise consultations (decisional balance, goal-setting, relapse prevention, problem-solving, exploration of activity options, social support), taking part in group counselling and behaviour-modification sessions (self-efficacy enhancement, problem-solving skills, relapse-prevention strategies), using PA diaries, and devising an action plan for PA performance can have a positive effect. A key concept is self-efficacy. In social cognitive theory, self-efficacy is described as an individual's belief in their ability to perform a particular behaviour in a variety of circumstances. Self-efficacy beliefs regarding the ability to exercise daily despite

Table 17.1 Barriers to maintaining adequate PA levels in the long term	
Intrapersonal	Physical condition
	Competing demands
	Work responsibilities
	Lack of time
	Lack of motivation
	Lack of interest
	Acceptance of sedentary lifestyle
Interpersonal	Social/family obligations
	Lack of social support
	Housework
	Caregiving responsibilities
Environmental	Inclement weather
	Distance
	Environmental resources/facilities
Organizational	Time of activity/scheduling
	Financial costs

barriers (bad weather, a lot of work, lack of time, health problems) predicts the adherence to recommended exercises. However, maintaining regular PA for months and years after phase II CR is a complex task and requires not only good baseline self-efficacy, but also the ability to self-regulate actions when rescheduling and reorganizing daily life. From this perspective, all staff members involved in multidisciplinary CR during the transition phase can help in identifying 'maintainers' and 'relapsers' with regard to PA.

How to prescribe and/or recommend regular physical activity after phase II cardiac rehabilitation

An individually prescribed programme (type, intensity, duration, frequency) based on the underlying cardiac condition and the current cardiorespiratory fitness level (assessed by direct testing) is the ideal approach to maximizing the benefits and minimizing the risks of PA. Similarly, identification of training goals and regular follow-up will help to establish better conditions for maintaining regular PA in daily activities in the long term.

When such a structured prescription is not available, patients at low risk of cardiac events should be recommended to participate in regular non-supervised leisure time PA. It should be mainly aerobic, at an intensity between the first and second ventilatory threshold and below the ischaemic/arrhythmic threshold, if known. Individuals should be encouraged to choose some activity that they enjoy and/or can include in their daily routine. Aerobic PA consists of movements of large muscle mass in a rhythmic manner for a sustained period. It includes everyday activity, leisure time activity, and exercise such as brisk walking, Nordic walking, hiking, jogging or running, cycling, cross-country skiing, aerobic dancing, skating, rowing, or swimming. Both moderate and vigorous aerobic exercise intensities can be recommended, although it is is necessary to distinguish between absolute and relative intensities. Absolute intensity is the amount of energy expended per minute of activity, assessed by oxygen uptake per unit of time or by metabolic equivalent (MET), while relative intensity refers to the level of effort required to perform an activity (Table 17.2). They may not correspond in cardiac patients with different fitness levels, and this should be taken into account when prescribing long-term PA protocols. The frequency of PA sessions should be at least three to five per week, preferably every day. Training volume (or dose) is the main driver for prescription, and it is recommended that individuals accumulate at least 30 min/day, 5 days/week of moderate intensity PA (i.e. 150 min/week), or 15 min/ day, 5 days/week of vigorous intensity PA (75 min/week), or a combination of both, performed in sessions lasting for at least 10 min.

Aerobic interval training and high-intensity training can also be considered in an individualized prescription. Resistance/strength training could also be associated with aerobic training in this scenario, with the following precautions.

(1) Target major muscle groups (agonist and antagonist).

(2) Include multi-joint or compound movements through the full range of motion of the joints.

(3) Avoid the Valsalva manoeuvre during exercise.

Table 17.2 Absolute and relative intensity levels for moderate and vigorous activities	
Moderate activity	
Examples: walking briskly, slow cycling, gardening, golf, tennis (doubles), ballroom dancing, water aerobics	Absolute intensity: 3–5.9 MET Relative intensity: • 64–76% of measured or estimated maximum HR • Borg scale score 12–13 Breathing is faster but compatible with speaking full sentences
Vigorous activity	
Examples: jogging, running, bicycling (>15 km/h, heavy gardening, swimming laps, tennis (singles)	Absolute intensity: ≥6 METs Relative intensity: • 77–93 % of measured or estimated maximum HR • Borg scale score 14–16 Breathing very hard and incompatible with carrying on a conversation comfortably

(4) Prescribe two or three sets of 8–12 repetitions at an intensity of 60–80% of the individual's one repetition maximum (1-RM) (i.e. the maximum load that can be lifted once) at a frequency of least two days a week. Older adults or very deconditioned individuals should start with one set of 10–15 repetitions at 60–70% 1-RM.

In the case of both fully structured or recommended PA activities after phase II CR, patients need to receive information about general examples of good PA practice (Box 17.1). In the case of participation in competitive sports, low-static and low-dynamic type of sports should be preferred [3].

Box 17.1 Suggestions for good physical activity practice

- Always include three periods in each PA session: warm-up, training and cool-down.
- Report any unusual symptoms such as chest pain, dizziness, dyspnoea, or palpitations during PA to the physician.
- No PA in cases of unusual asthenia, fever or viral syndrome.
- Ensure adequate hydration before, during, and after PA.
- Adapt the intensity of physical activity to the environmental conditions (temperature, humidity, altitude).
- Avoid smoking at all times, especially immediately before and after PA.
- Avoid a hot shower for 15 min after PA.
- Tailor the intensity of PA to the individual's current clinical physical capacity.
- Avoid any kind of drug abuse, doping, and/or additives with contents that are not fully known.

Regular medical follow-ups, including fitness assessments and patient education on how to deal with new or increased symptoms, are recommended in order to reduce CV events. Automatic external defibrillators should be available at facilities such as gyms or sport arenas when phase III CR patients participate in sports and other physical activities, and the staff should be trained in cardiopulmonary resuscitation.

Conclusion

The transition between phases II and III of CR poses specific issues and tasks regarding PA, and most of these need a tailored solution before patients return to primary care. Promoting continuing PA is a major challenge for modern CR programmes, but is also an essential opportunity for reducing CV events and re-hospitalizations. In the near future, digital health tools—based either online (eHealth) or on smart phone (mHealth), where patients record and monitor their exercise programme—could help to promote and maintain adherence in the long term.

References

1. Vanhees L, Rauch B, Piepoli M, et al. Importance of characteristics and modalities of physical activity and exercise in the management of cardiovascular health in individuals with cardiovascular disease (Part III). *Eur J Prev Cardiol* 2012; 19(6): 1333–56.

2. Piepoli MF, Hoes AW, Agewall S, et al. 2016 European Guidelines on cardiovascular disease prevention in clinical practice. The Sixth Joint Task Force of the European Society of Cardiology and Other Societies on Cardiovascular Disease Prevention in Clinical Practice. *Eur J Prev Cardiol* 2016; 23: NP1–96.

3. Börjesson M, Assanelli D, Carré F, et al. ESC Study Group of Sports Cardiology: recommendations for participation in leisure-time physical activity and competitive sports for patients with ischaemic heart disease. *Eur J Cardiovasc Prev Rehabil* 2006; 13: 137–49.

Further reading

Pratesi A, Baldasseroni S, Burgisser C, et al. Long-term functional outcomes after cardiac rehabilitation in older patients. Data from the Cardiac Rehabilitation in Advanced aGE: EXercise TRaining and Active follow-up (CR-AGE EXTRA) randomised study. *Eur J Prev Cardiol* 2019; 26: 1470–8.

Lunde P, Bye A, Bergland A, et al. Long-term follow-up with a smartphone application improves exercise capacity post cardiac rehabilitation: a randomized controlled trial. *Eur J Prev Cardiol* 2020; doi: 10.1177/2047487320905717.

Franklin BA, Thompson PD, Al-Zaiti SS, et al. Exercise-related acute cardiovascular events and potential deleterious adaptations following long-term exercise training: placing the risks into perspective—an update: a scientific statement from the American Heart Association. *Circulation* 2020; 141; e705–36.

Del Pozo-Cruz B, Carrick-Ranson G, Reading S, et al. The relationship between exercise dose and health-related quality of life with a phase III cardiac rehabilitation program. *Qual Life Res* 2018; 27: 993–8.

Chapter 18

Cardiopulmonary exercise test

Luca Moderato and Massimo Francesco Piepoli

Summary

Cardiopulmonary exercise testing (CPET) is a safe and reproducible diagnostic tool for the global assessment of cardiovascular (CV), ventilatory, and metabolic responses to exercise. It can be extremely useful for understanding the reasons for dyspnoea, fatigue, and exercise limitation, and for differentiating between cardiac and pulmonary disorders. CPET can also help the clinician to optimize the decision-making process and outcome prediction, especially in heart failure (HF) patients.

151

Introduction

CPET in HF patients was first described by Weber and colleagues in 1982 [1] as a non-invasive method for assessing the behaviour of the cardiopulmonary system during physical stress by analysing exhaled gases to measure minute ventilation, oxygen uptake, and CO_2 production. CPET provides a reproducible global assessment of the CV, ventilatory, and metabolic responses to exercise to obtain diagnostic and prognostic information. This tool enables the clinician to evaluate reasons for dyspnoea and fatigue and to differentiate pulmonary from cardiac disorders; it also allows optimization of the decision-making process and outcome prediction, and objectively determines targets for pharmacological and non-pharmacological therapies [2], especially in HF patients. Indications for CPET [3] are listed in Table 18.1.

Physiology of exercise

Peak exercise capacity is defined as 'the maximum ability of the CV system to deliver oxygen to muscles and of the muscles to extract oxygen from the blood'. Therefore exercise tolerance is mainly determined by three factors:

a) CV performance, including endothelial function of the peripheral arteries

b) pulmonary gas exchange

c) skeletal muscle metabolism.

In healthy individuals, exercise usually leads to an increase in HR and contractility; ventilation gradually increases, led by the rise of respiratory rate, and alveolar perfusion and ventilation (alveolar recruitment) take place. The rise in HR and contractility will achieve a plateau when maximal exercise capacity is reached. Respiratory capacity by

Table 18.1 Definition and normal values of CPET variables

Evaluation of exercise tolerance

  Determination of functional impairment or capacity (peak VO_2)

  Determination of exercise-limiting factors

Evaluation of undiagnosed exercise intolerance

  Assessing contribution of cardiac and pulmonary aetiology in coexisting disease

  Symptoms disproportionate to resting pulmonary and cardiac tests

  Unexplained dyspnoea when standard pulmonary function test is not diagnostic

Evaluation of patients with cardiovascular disease

  Functional evaluation and prognosis in patients with heart failure

  Selection for cardiac transplantation

  Exercise prescription and monitoring response to exercise training for cardiac rehabilitation (special circumstances, i.e. pacemakers)

Evaluation of patients with respiratory disease

  Functional impairment assessment

  Chronic obstructive pulmonary disease

  Establishing exercise limitation and assessing other potential contributing as occult heart disease

  Determination of magnitude of hypoxaemia and for O_2 prescription

Interstitial lung diseases

  Detection of early gas exchange abnormalities

  Overall assessment/monitoring of pulmonary gas exchange

  Determination of magnitude of hypoxaemia and for O_2 prescription

  Determination to response to potentially toxic therapy

Pulmonary vascular disease (careful risk-benefit analysis required)

Cystic fibrosis

Exercise-induced bronchospasm

Specific clinical applications

  Pre-operative evaluation

  Lung resectional surgery

  Evaluation for lung, heart-lung transplantation

Reproduced from Task Force of the Italian Working Group on Cardiac Rehabilitation and Prevention (Gruppo Italiano di Cardiologia Riabilitativa e Prevenzione, GICR); Working Group on Cardiac Rehabilitation and Exercise Physiology of the European Society of Cardiology, Piepoli MF, et al. Statement on cardiopulmonary exercise testing in chronic heart failure due to left ventricular dysfunction: recommendations for performance and interpretation Part II: How to perform cardiopulmonary exercise testing in chronic heart failure. *Eur J Cardiovasc Prev Rehabil* 2006;13(3):300-311. doi:10.1097/00149831-200606000-00003 with permission from SAGE.

far exceeds the demands of peak exercise (pulmonary reserve). This is the reason why exercise capacity in healthy individuals is rarely affected by respiratory limitation.

The Fick equation

The Fick equation is of key importance for the evaluation of the utility of functional exercise testing with gas exchange measurement. According to the Fick equation, VO_2 equals cardiac output multiplied by the arterial oxygen content minus the mixed venous oxygen content:

$$VO_2 = (SV \times HR) \times (CaO_2 - CvO_2)$$

where SV is stroke volume, HR is heart rate, CaO_2 is the arterial oxygen content, and CvO_2 is the mixed venous oxygen content.

Oxygen uptake is usually normalized for body weight and expressed in units of $mlO_2/kg/min$. One MET is defined as the resting oxygen uptake and equals 3.5 ml/kg/min.

At maximal exercise, the Fick equation is expressed as:

$$VO_{2max} = (SV_{max} \times HR_{max}) \times (CaO_{2max} - CvO_{2max})$$

which reflects the maximal ability of uptake, transport, and use of oxygen, and defines the patient's functional aerobic capacity. In healthy people, VO_2 reaches a plateau at near-maximal exercise (Figure 18.1). This plateau has traditionally been

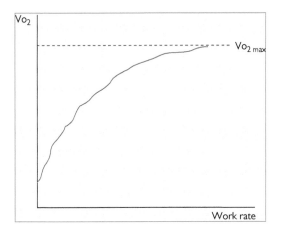

Figure 18.1 Estimation of maximal oxygen uptake.

Reproduced from Statement on cardiopulmonary exercise testing in chronic heart failure due to left ventricular dysfunction: recommendations for performance and interpretation. Part I: definition of cardiopulmonary exercise testing parameters for appropriate use in chronic heart failure. Task Force of the Italian Working Group on Cardiac Rehabilitation Prevention; Working Group on Cardiac Rehabilitation and Exercise Physiology of the European Society of Cardiology, Piepoli MF, Corrà U, Agostoni PG, et al. *Eur J Cardiovasc Prev Rehabil* 2006 Apr; 13(2): 150–64 with permission from SAGE Publishing.

used as the best evidence for $VO_{2\,max}$ [4]. However, in the clinical setting, a clear plateau is often not reached because of the occurrence of symptoms limiting exercise capacity; consequently, peak VO_2 is often used as a surrogate for $VO_{2\,max}$.

$VO_{2\,max}$ has become the preferred measure of cardiorespiratory fitness and is the most important measurement made during functional exercise testing.

How to perform a cardiopulmonary exercise test

Pre-test consideration

Several methods exist for measuring ventilation and respiratory gas during exercise. Most clinical systems rely on breath-by-breath analysis techniques. A non-rebreathing valve is connected to a mouthpiece to prevent mixing of inspired and expired air. Oxygen and CO_2 gas analysers are usually incorporated in a metabolic cart designed for functional testing.

Respiratory volumes are measured by integrating the air flow over time of inspiration and expiration. Average minute volumes are derived from the breath-by-breath data multiplied by the respiratory rate.

The exercise is performed on a bicycle or a treadmill (NB: as cycling is a non-weight-bearing exercise, peak oxygen uptake is systematically 10–20% lower than during treadmill exercise). Cycle ergometry has become more popular for obese patients and for patients with orthopaedic limitations or balance instability. Furthermore, data recorded during a bicycle test are less prone to movement artefacts and allow a more accurate analysis in the case of a ramp protocol. Many different protocols are used for functional testing. The purpose of the test and the fitness level, age, and body surface area (BSA) of the patient determine the choice of protocol. The rate of workload progression can be chosen arbitrarily, although a less steep ramp is recommended to optimize gas registration and avoid premature exhaustion. The optimal exercise duration is considered to be between 8 and 12 min [5,6].

Patient collaboration is essential to optimize the clinical and diagnostic value of CPET. Patients must be adequately instructed, in order to achieve the best effort possible relative to their condition (Box 18.1).

The metabolic cart must be calibrated before every session in order to maintain accuracy of gas and ventilation measurements. Spirometry is then performed to

---

Box 18.1 General indications for cardiopulmonary exercise testing

- Patient consent and collaboration.
- Protocol selection and explanation of test protocol.
- History and clinical examination.
- Assessment of comorbidites (e.g. orthopaedic limitations).
- Anthropometric measurements: weight, height, body mass index, body surface area.
- Resting ECG, BP, and oxygen saturation.
- Pre-test spirometry.

evaluate the resting pulmonary function. Forced spirometry manoeuvres including forced expiratory volume in 1 sec (FEV_1), forced vital capacity (FVC) and peak expiratory flow (PEF) are required to substantiate the extent of any respiratory limitation during exercise. Maximum voluntary ventilation (the maximum volume of air ventilated in 60 sec) and breathing reserve (BR), derived from CPET, can aid in the determination of normal respiratory function. An ECG monitor and a blood pressure (BP) monitor are attached to the patient, and a facial mask or a mouthpiece is used to measure ventilation and gas exchange.

Conducting the test

The test should be started with 1–2 min registration during rest, followed by 2–3 min warm-up (pedalling or walking without resistance). The pedalling rate should be 60–70 rev/min throughout the test. The test should be stopped if 60 rev/min can no longer be maintained.

BP should be recorded at rest and every 2 min thereafter or during the final minute of each exercise stage in non-ramp protocols; perceived ratings of dyspnoea and fatigue (Borg scale) should be recorded at the end of the test in order to differentiate between dyspnoea and muscular fatigue as the reason for terminating the exercise. The ECG should be carefully monitored to check signs of ischaemia or the occurrence of arrhythmias [6].

CPET should be performed as a symptom-limited test, i.e. it should be stopped when the patient is unable to maintain a minimal rate of pedalling due to exhaustion or if any of the following indications to stop the examination occurs:

a) significant arrhythmia (bursts of ventricular tachycardia, sustained ventricular tachycardia)
b) second- or third-degree heart block
c) decrease of systolic BP (i.e. any decrease) during heavy exercise
d) ST segment depression >2 mm
e) patient distress
f) chest pain suggestive of cardiac ischaemia
g) loss of coordination
h) near-syncope, dizziness, or confusion
i) symptomatic severe hypoxaemia (oxygen saturation <80%).

When the exercise protocol is stopped, the patient is asked to continue pedalling or walking slowly for 1 min; then 4–5 min of further recording are usually performed. It is important to ask the patient at the end of the test which symptom limited their effort most: leg fatigue, dyspnoea, or any other reason.

Interpreting the results of cardiopulmonary exercise tests

Test analysis is generally started with identification of the first lactate threshold or the ventilatory threshold (VT). Several methods are available (Figure 18.2):

- Ventilatory equivalents: this method involves the simultaneous analysis of several variables: VE/VO_2, VE/VCO_2, $PETO_2$, and $PETCO_2$. VT is defined as

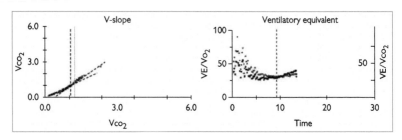

Figure 18.2 Estimation of the anaerobic treshold according to modified V-slope method and the ventilatory equivalent.

Reproduced from Statement on cardiopulmonary exercise testing in chronic heart failure due to left ventricular dysfunction: recommendations for performance and interpretation. Part I: definition of cardiopulmonary exercise testing parameters for appropriate use in chronic heart failure. Task Force of the Italian Working Group on Cardiac Rehabilitation Prevention; Working Group on Cardiac Rehabilitation and Exercise Physiology of the European Society of Cardiology, Piepoli MF, Corrà U, Agostoni PG, et al. *Eur J Cardiovasc Prev Rehabil* 2006 Apr; 13(2): 150–64 with permission from SAGE Publishing.

the VO_2 value at which VE/VO_2 and $PETO_2$ reach a minimum and thereafter begin to rise consistently, coinciding with an unchanged VE/VCO_2 and $PETCO_2$ (Figure 18.3).

- V-slope: the ventilatory threshold (VT) is identified as the VO_2 at which the change in slope of the relationship between VCO_2 and VO_2 occurs.

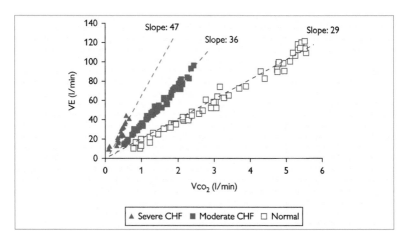

Figure 18.3 Relationship between ventilation (VE) and CO_2 production (VE/VCO_2 slope): CHF, chronic heart failure.

Reproduced from Statement on cardiopulmonary exercise testing in chronic heart failure due to left ventricular dysfunction: recommendations for performance and interpretation. Part I: definition of cardiopulmonary exercise testing parameters for appropriate use in chronic heart failure. Task Force of the Italian Working Group on Cardiac Rehabilitation Prevention; Working Group on Cardiac Rehabilitation and Exercise Physiology of the European Society of Cardiology, Piepoli MF, Corrà U, Agostoni PG, et al. *Eur J Cardiovasc Prev Rehabil* 2006 Apr; 13(2): 150–64 with permission from SAGE Publishing.

- Modified V-slope: this method determines the point of change in the slope of the relationship between VCO_2 and VO_2 and defines the VO_2 above which VCO_2 increases faster than VO_2 without hyperventilation [7].

Oxygen consumption (VO_2)

Oxygen consumption is the volume of oxygen extracted from the air inhaled during pulmonary ventilation in a unit of time, and is expressed in ml/min, usually standardized for BSA and expressed as ml/kg/min.

The normal values depend on several factors, such as age, sex, weight, height, physical activity level, genetic variability, and ethnicity. Various equations are used to predict the normal values of oxygen uptake, but the one proposed by Wasserman et al. [4] is used most frequently.

VO_2 at peak exercise is the most important parameter for evaluating disease severity in patients with HF, pulmonary hypertension, hypertrophic cardiomyopathy, chronic obstructive pulmonary disease (COPD), and restrictive pulmonary disease, in addition to physical fitness level [8–10]. A normal value for oxygen uptake is considered >20.0 ml/kg/min, and values <10ml/kg/min predict poor prognosis [11].

Peak VO_2 and oxygen uptake at VT are influenced by genetic predisposition, disease, amount of exercise taken, and aerobic training type. A normal VO_2 at VT for adults is about 40–65% of predicted VO_2 [11]. The VT value is important for individualized prescription of exercise, as well as for diagnosis of anaemia, physical fitness, myopathies, and cardiomyopathies [12].

Pulmonary ventilation (VE)

Ventilation is expressed in litres per minute. It is determined as the respiratory rate mutiplied by the volume of air exhaled at every cycle (tidal volume). At rest, 7–9 l/min are ventilated, but in athletes that value can reach 200 l/min at maximal exertion [1].

Ventilation increases continuously during progressive effort on CPET until the respiratory compensation point (RCP), when the body increases CO_2 output in order to compensate for the accumulation of lactic acid (second lactate threshold).

Periodic (or oscillatory) ventilation is defined as an oscillatory pattern of ventilation, which persists in ≥60% of the effort with an amplitude ≥15% compared with mean resting values. It reflects disease severity and relates to worse prognosis in patients with HF [10–14].

Respiratory exchange ratio (RER)

RER is the ratio of CO_2 production to O_2 consumption (VCO_2/VO_2). It is the best non-invasive indicator of exercise intensity, as values >1.10 have been accepted as a parameter of maximal exercise [8–10].

VE/VCO$_2$ slope (ventilatory efficiency)

This is the slope obtained from the relationship between VE and VCO_2 (VE/VCO_2 slope) and quantifies the amount of ventilation required to eliminate 1 L of CO_2. VE/VCO_2 can be determined up to either the respiratory compensation point or the maximal value. It is important to know which type of measurement was adopted when the slope is used for prognostic purposes (Figure 18.3).

VE/VCO$_2$ is a very sensitive, although non-specific, marker of gas exchange and can be altered by pre- or post-capillary changes as well as by disorders affecting gas diffusion. VE/VCO$_2$ is a major exercise-related risk marker in CHF, even more powerful than peak VO$_2$ [15]. In fact, an elevation of VE/VCO$_2$ is frequently observed in patients with chronic HF (Figure 18.3), and can be used to evaluate the effectiveness of a number of treatments including exercise training (ET), cardiac resynchronization therapy, and heart transplantation [16–20]. The normal value should be <30.0, and values of 36–44 and >45.0 are respectively moderately and severely elevated and predictive of poor prognosis in HF patients [11].

Oxygen pulse (VO$_2$/HR)

Oxygen pulse is the ratio of VO$_2$ to HR (Figure 18.4). It reflects the amount of oxygen extracted per heart beat and has been used as an estimator of stroke volume during exercise. The oxygen pulse normally increases with incremental exercise because of the increases in both SV and oxygen extraction and then reaches a plateau.

A low flat O$_2$ pulse increase can be interpreted as resulting from reduced SV and/or as a failure of further skeletal muscle oxygen extraction. A decrease in the oxygen pulse during the stress test is a sign of exercise-induced ischaemia (decrease of SV due to wall motion abnormalities in relation to ischaemia). Therefore a low oxygen pulse may reflect deconditioning, increasing mitral regurgitation during exercise, or ischaemia [8–21].

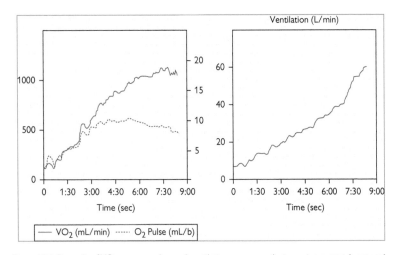

Figure 18.4 Example of VO$_2$, oxygen pulse, and ventilation responses during an incremental protocol on a cycle ergometer (20W/min, ramp) in a 70-year-old man referred for chest discomfort. Both VO$_2$ and oxygen pulse flatten, while ventilation continues to rise without any evident point of inflection.

Reproduced from Belardinelli, Romualdo et al. Cardiopulmonary exercise testing is more accurate than ECG-stress testing in diagnosing myocardial ischemia in subjects with chest pain. *International Journal of Cardiology*, Volume 174, Issue 2, 337–342 with permission from Elsevier.

Blood pressure response

As exercise intensity increases, the flow-mediated vasodilatation and initial decrease of systolic BP is soon overcome by the continuously increasing cardiac output and systolic BP until the end of the stress test. Diastolic BP typically remains constant or may decrease slightly if left-heart function keeps up with the increases in cardiac output. Abnormal patterns of BP response include excessive rise (dysregulation of BP control), reduced rise (decreased left-ventricular function), or a fall (ischaemia, outflow tract obstruction or aortic stenosis). A fall in BP despite increasing workload is an important indication for terminating the exercise [10–20].

Heart rate

In healthy subjects, HR increases almost linearly with increasing VO_2. This is mediated initially by a decrease in parasympathetic activity (vagal withdrawal) and subsequently by sympathetic stimulation. Achievement of age-predicted values for maximal HR during exercise is often used as a reflection of maximal or near maximal effort; however it should not be misunderstood as an indication for stress test termination. Furthermore, variation of maximal HR compared with theoretical age-predicted values is huge (± 20 bpm) and can also be influenced by medication and sympathetic desensitization in HF.

The value of HR at VT is of outmost importance for aerobic exercise prescription.

HR recovery (HRR) in the first minute after the end of the test is an important prognostic indicator, with poor prognosis for HF patients with values <12 bpm [11–22].

End-tidal CO_2 partial pressure ($PETCO_2$)

$PETCO_2$ reflects ventilation–perfusion mismatch within the pulmonary system and, indirectly, cardiac function. Its value ranges from 36 to 42 mmHg, with 3- to 8-mmHg elevations during moderate intensity exercise, reaching a maximal value with a subsequent drop, due to VE increase, characterizing the RCP. Abnormal values may indicate disease severity in patients with HF, hypertrophic cardiomyopathy, pulmonary HTN, COPD, and restrictive pulmonary disease [8,23,24].

Breathing reserve (VE/MVV)

BR is the difference between maximal ventilation during exercise (VE) and maximum voluntary ventilation (MVV) at rest. Since direct measurement of MVV is difficult (over a period of only 15 sec), it is generally calculated on the basis of FEV_1:

$$MVV = FEV_1 \times 40.$$

Normal values for BR are >0.20 or >10 L. It is useful in the differential diagnosis of dyspnoea.

$\Delta VO_2/\Delta WR$ relationship

This is the relationship between VO_2 (ml/min) and the workload (WR) slope during a ramp protocol. Since there is a linear increase in cardiac output (SV × HR) with workload, a low $\Delta VO_2/\Delta WR$ relationship reflects a decrease in SV, assuming that

Table 18.2 Definition and normal values of CPET variables

CPET variables	Definition	Values
VO_2	Describes functional capacity reduced in all diseases according to severity Prognosis indicator	Normal: >20 ml/kg/min Mildly reduced: 16–20 ml/kg/min Moderately reduced: 10.0–15.9 ml/kg/min Severely reduced: <10 ml/kg/min
VO_2%	Describes functional capacity relative to predicted normal values	Normal, >100% of predicted Mild reduction: 99–75% of predicted Moderate reduction:75–50% of predicted Severe reduction: <50% of predicted
VE/VCO_2 slope	Describes pulmonary ventilation and perfusion Increased in HF, PHTN Mildly increased in pulmonary disease Prognosis indicator	Normal: <30.0 Mildly elevated: 30.0–35.9 Moderately elevated: 36.0–44.9 Severely elevated: >45.0 (Arena Classification)
Exercise oscillatory ventilation (EOV)	Present in HF Predicts poor prognosis	Present: must persist for 60% of the exercise test with amplitude ≥15% Absent
Breathing reserve (VE/MVV)	Differential diagnosis of dyspnoea from pulmonary origin	Normal values: >0.20
End-tidal CO_2 partial pressure ($PETCO_2$)	Reflects ventilation–perfusion Indicates disease severity in patients with HF, HCM, PHTN, COPD, and restrictive pulmonary disease	Normal values Resting $PETCO_2$ >33.0 mmHg or 3–8 mmHg increase during ET Abnormal values Resting $PETCO_2$ <33.0 mm Hg and or <3 mmHg increase during ET
Oxygen pulse (VO_2/HR)	Estimates stroke volume	Usually normalized to BSA In healthy subjects increases during exercise Early plateau may suggest onset of myocardial ischaemia
Blood pressure	Usually systolic BP increases and diastolic BP decreases during exercise	Normal: rise in systolic BP Mild alteration: flat systolic BP response Severe alteration: drop in systolic BP
Respiratory exchange ratio (RER)	Expresses the ratio of CO_2 production to O_2 consumption (VCO_2/VO_2)	Values >1.10 are a parameter of maximal exercise

PHTN, pulmonary hypertension; HCM, hypertrophic cardiomyopathy chronotropic response is adequate. Therefore it is useful in the diagnosis of left ventricular dysfunction during exertion similar to an oxygen pulse. Its normal value for adults is >9–11 ml/min/Watt.

Conclusion

CPET is the most accurate method for assessing the exercise capacity of patients referred to CR programmes. It enables determination of the maximum exercise capacity, identification of exercise limitation factors, and evaluation of symptoms triggered by physical exercise. Interpretation of the test must take all variables in to consideration (Table 18.2) as their combined analysis may better stratify the patient.

CPET should be performed on admission to the CR programme, in order to optimize the prescription of exercise intensity and duration, and at discharge, but can also be repeated when a global reassessment is needed.

References

1. Weber KT, Kinasewitz GT, Janicki JS, Fishman AP. Oxygen utilization and ventilation during exercise in patients with chronic cardiac failure. *Circulation* 1982; 65:1213–23.
2. Guazzi M, Arena R, Halle M, et al. 2016 focused update: clinical recommendations for cardiopulmonary exercise testing data assessment in specific patient populations. *Circulation* 2016; 133: e694–711.
3. Piepoli MF, Corrà U, Agostoni PG, et al. Statement on cardiopulmonary exercise testing in chronic heart failure due to left ventricular dysfunction: recommendations for performance and interpretation. Part I: definition of cardiopulmonary exercise testing parameters for appropriate use in chronic heart failure. Task Force of the Italian Working Group on Cardiac Rehabilitation Prevention; Working Group on Cardiac Rehabilitation and Exercise Physiology of the European Society of Cardiology. *Eur J Cardiovasc Prev Rehabil* 2006; 13: 150–64.
4. Wasserman K, Hansen JE, Sue DY, et al. *Principles of Exercise Testing Aad Interpretation* (4th edn). Philadelphia, PA: Lippincott, Williams & Wilkins, 2005.
5. Luks AM, Glenny RW, Robertson HT. *Introduction to Cardiopulmonary Exercise Testing.* New York: Springer, 2013.
6. Buchfuhrer MJ, Hansen JE, Robinson TE, et al. Optimizing the exercise protocol for cardiopulmonary assessment. *J Appl Physiol* 1983; 55: 1558–64.
7. Piepolo MF, Corrà U, Agostoni PG, et al. Statement on cardiopulmonary exercise testing in chronic heart failure due to left ventricular dysfunction: recommendations for performance and interpretation. Part II: How to perform cardiopulmonary exercise testing in chronic heart failure. *Eur J Cardiovasc Prev Rehabil* 2006; 13: 300–311.
8. Guazzi M, Adams V, Conraads V, et al. European Association for Cardiovascular Prevention and Rehabilitation; American Heart Association. EACPR/AHA Scientific Statement. Clinical recommendations for cardiopulmonary exercise testing data assessment in specific patient populations. *Circulation* 2012; 126: 2261–74.
9. Sorajja P, Allison T, Hayes C, et al. Prognostic utility of metabolic exercise testing in minimally symptomatic patients with obstructive hypertrophic cardiomyopathy. *Am J Cardiol* 2012; 109: 1494–8.
10. Task Force of the Italian Working Group on Cardiac Rehabilitation and Prevention (Gruppo Italiano di Cardiologia Riabilitativa e Prevenzione, GICR); Working Group on Cardiac Rehabilitation and Exercise Physiology of the European Society of Cardiology. Statement on cardiopulmonary exercise testing in chronic heart failure due to left ventricular dysfunction: recommendations for performance and interpretation. Part III: Interpretation of cardiopulmonary exercise testing in chronic heart failure and future applications. *Eur J Cardiovasc Prev Rehabil* 2006; 13: 485–94.

11. Guazzi M, Bandera F, Ozemek F, et al. Cardiopulmonary exercise testing. *J Am Coll Cardiol* 2017; 70: 1618–36.

12. Wasserman K, Whipp BJ. Exercise physiology in health and disease. *Am Rev Resp Dis* 1975; 112: 219–49.

13. Herdy AH, Uhnlerdorf D. Reference values for cardiopulmonary exercise testing for sedentary and active men and women. *Arq Bras Cardiol* 2011; 96: 54–9.

14. Corrà U, Giordano A, Bosimini E, et al. Oscillatory ventilation during exercise in patients with chronic heart failure: clinical correlates and prognostic implications. *Chest* 2002; 121: 1572–80.

15. Mezzani A, Giordano A, Komici K, Corrà U. Different determinants of ventilatory inefficiency at different stages of reduced ejection fraction chronic heart failure natural history. *J Am Heart Assoc* 2017; 6: e 005278.

16. Sullivan MJ, Higginbotham MB, Cobb FR. Increased exercise ventilation in patients with chronic heart failure: intact ventilatory control despite hemodynamic and pulmonary abnormalities. *Circulation* 1988; 77: 552–9.

17. Guazzi M, Tumminello G, Di Marco F, Fiorentini C, The effects of phosphodiesterase-5 inhibition with sildenafil on pulmonary hemodynamics and diffusion capacity, exercise ventilatory efficiency, and oxygen uptake kinetics in chronic heart failure. *J Am Coll Cardiol* 2004; 44: 2339–48.

18. Malfatto G, Facchini M, Branzi G, et al. Reverse ventricular remodeling and improved functional capacity after ventricular resynchronization in advanced heart failure. *Ital Heart J* 2005; 6; 578–83.

19. Carter R, Al-Rawas O, Stevenson A, et al. Exercise responses following heart transplantation: 5 year follow-up. *Scott Med J* 2006; 51: 6–14.

20. Piepoli MF, Corrà U, Agostoni PG, et al. Statement on cardiopulmonary exercise testing in chronic heart failure due to left ventricular dysfunction: recommendations for performance and interpretation. Part I: definition of cardiopulmonary exercise testing parameters for appropriate use in chronic heart failure. *Eur J Cardiovasc Prev Rehabil* 2006; 13: 150–64.

21. Belardinelli R, Lacalaprice F, Tiano L, et al. Cardiopulmonary exercise testing is more accurate than ECG-stress testing in diagnosing myocardial ischemia in subjects with chest pain. *Int J Cardiol* 2014; 174: 337–42.

22. Qiu S, Cai X, Sun Z, et al. Heart rate recovery and risk of cardiovascular events and all-cause mortality: a meta-analysis of prospective cohort studies. *J Am Heart Assoc* 2017; 6: e005505.

23. Sorajja P, Allison T, Hayes C, et al. Prognostic utility of metabolic exercise testing in minimally symptomatic patients with obstructive hypertrophic cardiomyopathy. *Am J Cardiol* 2012; 109: 1494–8.

24. Torchio R, Guglielmo M, Giardino R, et al. Exercise ventilatory inefficiency and mortality in patients with chronic obstructive pulmonary disease undergoing surgery for non-small-cell lung cancer. *Eur J Cardiothorac Surg* 2010; 38: 14–19.

Further reading

Corrà U, Agostoni PG, Anker SD, et al. Role of cardiopulmonary exercise testing in clinical stratification in heart failure. A position paper from the Committee on Exercise Physiology and Training of the Heart Failure, Association of the European Society of Cardiology. *Eur J Heart Fail* 2018; 20, 3–15.

Sarullo FM, Fazio G, Brusca I, et al. Cardiopulmonary exercise testing in patients with chronic heart failure: prognostic comparison from peak VO_2 and VE/VCO_2 slope. *Open Cardiovasc Med J* 2010; 4: 127–34.

Chapter 19

Technological issues

Martijn Scherrenberg, Cindel Bonneux, Ines Frederix, and Paul Dendale

Summary

Technology has become increasingly important in cardiac rehabilitation (CR). New technologies, such as smartwatches, have changed the landscape of real-time monitoring of ambulatory patients. Implementation of new technology is always accompanied by issues of concern. Relevant examples are inter-operability and data protection. However, new technologies mainly offer new opportunities such as improvements in tele-rehabilitation (teleCR), persuasive design and big data analysis.

Introduction

In the last decade, technology has increasingly been used in CR. Newer technologies, such as applications on mobile devices, allow a wider range of telehealth possibilities. Heart rate (HR) monitoring is already part of standard care in most CR programmes to ensure that patients exercise at the recommended HR [1]. In recent years hip-worn accelerometers have often been used to assess physical activity (PA) and sedentary time for cardiovascular (CV) patients. A number of teleCR studies have used these devices to monitor the PA of patients at home and to provide feedback to them about their activity pattern [2,3]. However, smartphones and, more recently, smartwatches are gradually replacing accelerometers for activity tracking. Wrist-worn devices are capable of monitoring more than just PA. They can monitor HR, energy expenditure (EE), steps, and distance travelled [4,5]. Future possibilities for smartwatch use are innumerable, with the opportunity of measuring oxygen saturation, blood glucose, and cardiac arrhythmia [5]. Important technological issues in the use of technology in CR are inter-operability and big data. Inter-operable systems will result in significantly lower implementation and integration costs. Big data, which are extremely large datasets that cannot be analysed using traditional data-processing methods [6], can be collected from mobile phone applications, wearable technology, social media, environmental and lifestyle-related factors, etc. Artificial intelligence (AI) is being used to process this data in order to improve the quality of patient care, improve cost-effectiveness, and facilitate precision CV medicine [6]. In this chapter we provide an overview of established and new technologies in cardiac telemedicine and rehabilitation. We also present important technological issues that can arise from the use of technology and discuss barriers to implementation.

Monitoring in cardiac rehabilitation

Collection of data

The best way of categorizing the different technologies that can be used in CR is by the data types that are collected [7]. An important difference in data collection is whether active patient engagement is required or there is a passive transmission of data. Most of the current technologies used in CR require active patient engagement. Examples of data where patient engagement is necessary are therapy adherence and the description of symptoms.

Innovations such as biosensors can contribute to a more passive way of data collection and therefore decrease patient dropout. Wearable data is probably the most useful as it allows individuals or caregivers to be informed about the effects of patient actions or treatments or their underlying clinical status [8]. Ideally, the data obtained can be the input for decision support systems and even built-in therapies using automatic or semi-automatic feedback loops [8].

Telemonitoring is traditionally defined as synchronous or asynchronous. In synchronous telemonitoring, the health information is delivered in real time and enables live discussion between patients and health professionals. In contrast, asynchronous telemedicine refers to the 'store-and-forward' technique. Patients or health professionals collect medical history, images, and pathology reports, and then send them to a specialist physician for diagnostic and treatment decisions [9].

Heart rate monitoring

HR monitoring devices have been available for many years. In the past, they were mainly used by athletes to monitor their development and performance [7]. More recently, with the emergence of smartwatches, HR monitoring has shifted from chest-strap to wrist-worn devices for continuous monitoring not only during exercise but also during rest.

The advantage of these devices is that both types can be used during hospital-based phase II CR programmes and in home-based phase III programmes. It is well known that HR monitoring is important during exercise training (ET). During a comprehensive CR programme, HR monitoring is used to assess the patient's individual exercise intensity [10].

The use of wearable HR monitors offers many opportunities within CR but also presents some interesting challenges. Firstly, the question remains as to whether the collection of massive quantities of data is significantly contributing to better clinical care [11]. Furthermore, recent European legislation about privacy and data collection raise important challenges. For example, which entities or individuals are responsible for this data and how it is handled?

Currently, there are still concerns about the accuracy of wearable HR monitors in daily clinical use. Wang et al. [12] concluded that none of the wrist-worn HR monitors that they tested achieved the accuracy of a chest-strap monitor. In general, the accuracy of wrist-worn monitors was best at rest and diminished with exercise. This could present a problem during CR where cardiac patients rely on these monitors to stay within physician-recommended safe HR thresholds during rehabilitation and exercise [12].

Tracking activity

The first device used for tracking activity was the pedometer [13]. However, issues such as data accuracy, reliability, and validity may have slowed its adoption for use in research [7,14]. Accelerometers measure the frequency and intensity of (tri)axial movement over time [15]. They are used in smartphones, smartwatches, and even implantable cardiac devices. Research has demonstrated that using these wearable activity monitors results in an increase in daily activity, lower body mass index, and even lower blood pressure [15].

As with HR monitoring, there are both opportunities and challenges in the use of activity tracker devices. They can provide positive feedback mechanisms to motivate patients and can also use goal-setting and reminders to increase the patient's adherence. However, one of the main problems is that most activity trackers are not extensively validated in healthy individuals or CV patients. Furthermore, activity trackers still have difficulties in assessing non-walking daily activities [16]. Therefore, more research into the accuracy of these trackers in a variety of sports activities is needed. However, the Telerehab III study [17] demonstrated that an accelerometer can be used in an effective way for teleCR in cardiac patients.

New trends: smartwatches and activity trackers

Smartwatches and activity trackers have entirely changed the landscape of HR monitoring and activity tracking. They have made both activity tracking and HR monitoring accessible to a larger population. One of the advantages of accelerometer-based smartwatches is that they use a three-axis accelerometer [18]. Thus the wearable device can be used to estimate the type of movement, count steps, calculate EE and energy intensity, and estimate sleep patterns [18].

Accuracy can be even higher with the addition of gyroscopes, magnetometers, barometers, and altimeters to the three-axis accelerometer. Most new smartphones and wearable devices use an inertial measurement unit. This calculates orientation using a combination of measurements by an accelerometer, a gyroscope, and a magnetometer [19].

Photoplethysmography (PPG) is a recently developed technology that is incorporated in wearable devices. It uses an optical technique to measure HR by detecting changes in blood volume beneath the skin. Currently, PPG lacks good accuracy because of signal noise produced by movement, ambient light, and tissue compression [20]. It is expected that in the future a combination of PPG and gyroscopes or accelerometers will be used to create algorithms for better HR measurements [21].

However, it is important to remain critical about the PPG technique because previous research has demonstrated that it is liable to poor accuracy during activities with increased physical exertion or involving repetitive contractions of the forearm skeletal muscles [22]. One of the disadvantages of current wrist-worn activity trackers is that there is evidence of systematic bias in the measurement of moderate to vigorous PA [23].

Haemodynamics monitoring in heart failure patients

Recently there has been an increasing amount of research on the development of technologies that can help to identify the first signs of HF decompensation [24]. HF decompensation is preceded by an increase in ventricular filling pressures and subsequently pulmonary oedema [25]. Early detection of these signs with remote dielectric sensing (ReDS) and bioimpedance enables early intervention to prevent decompensation [7].

ReDS is a technology based on electromagnetic energy which measures lung oedema concentration non-invasively [26]. It uses the differences in tissue dielectric properties to provide a numerical measurement of the degree of pulmonary congestion which correlates well with computed tomography results. In practice, these measurements are performed using a wearable vest. Future developments will make practical use even easier. Preliminary data on reduction in HF admissions have been promising, but additional experience is needed before ReDS data can be incorporated into standard clinical practice [7].

Another technology that can be used to detect HF decompensation is the wearable bioimpedance monitor. These devices measure transthoracic impedance by the application of a surface electrode. The research suggested that the degree of bioimpedance is inversely correlated with the level of intrathoracic fluid. These changes precede any standard clinical parameters and therefore may early detect decompensation [27].

Bioimpedance monitoring has the potential to be applied in a wearable non-invasive device to monitor pulmonary fluid status [28]. Possible future developments are employing bioimpedance for volume management and optimization of goal-directed medical therapy. However, a major disadvantage of bioimpedance technology is its low specificity [29].

Digital health

Digital health is a topic of great interest in CR. The use of mobile phone applications can make secondary prevention more personalized and can overcome current barriers to accessing CR. Therefore we will describe two important ways of using mobile health interventions to increase patient motivation and adherence [30].

Persuasive design in cardiac rehabilitation applications

Persuasive design deals with the attitude and behaviour change of users. As such, it can encourage new behaviours, modify existing behaviours, or reinforce current attitudes [31]. In this context, persuasive system design offers a way of addressing challenges to behaviour change, i.e. helping patients adopting a healthier lifestyle.

At the design level, persuasive techniques can be integrated into the visual elements of the application that can be seen by patients. At the application level, persuasion can be achieved through intelligibility, personalization, and tailoring of the components of the rehabilitation programme [32]. Evaluating the effectiveness of persuasive design is mostly done implicitly, for example by measuring patients' adherence to treatment. A multidisciplinary crossover study using a comprehensive patient-tailored application to support cardiac teleCR demonstrated that the persuasive design techniques integrated into the application and tailored goals for PA were effective in motivating patients to reach their teleCR targets [32].

Shared decision-making applications

Shared decision-making (SDM) is an approach that combines the available clinical evidence and the patient's personal values, preferences, goals, and context to reach a firmly based decision [33]. In an SDM process, the patient and caregiver have equally important roles: the expertise of the caregiver is considered as important as the patient's preferences [34].

Various initiatives have been undertaken to improve the uptake of SDM in practice, including advocacy for SDM in CV guidelines [35,36] and the availability of more digital aids to support decision-making [37]. Despite all these initiatives, there are numerous barriers preventing patients and caregivers from adopting SDM [38,39]. Thus, SDM has not been widely implemented in clinical practice [40].

Future directions

Big data analysis and artificial intelligence

Big data analytics is one of the buzzwords of the last decade. In the past, prediction models were developed on the basis of a small number of specified variables. The problem with these models is that they lack precision. They perform reasonably well on the population level, but not at the individual patient level [41]. Big data provides the opportunity to perform predictions ranging from mortality to patient-reported outcomes to resource utilization, and thus could be more clinically actionable [42]. The hallmark of big data is combining disparate data sources [42]. The use of mobile technology will increase the amount of data that can be analysed using AI. For example, data from wearables, biosensors, imaging, environmental data, information on social media networks, and more might be used to create more accurate predictions and tailored treatment recommendations [42].

The collection of big data is one thing but its analysis is another, and new tools are needed. AI techniques, such as machine learning, deep learning, and cognitive computing, will play a critical role in the evolution of CR and precision medicine [43]. AI is defined as the 'theory and development of computer systems able to perform tasks normally requiring human intelligence' [44]. Deep machine learning mimics the human brain by using large high-quality datasets to create layers of neural networks to generate automated predictions, interpret image data, and develop pattern recognition [43,45]. The ultimate goal of AI in cardiac healthcare is to help cardiologists make better diagnoses, have better therapy choices, and improve workflow, productivity, cost-effectiveness, and ultimately patient outcomes [46]. AI has already been used in automated predictions of CVD risk scores and HF diagnosis.

Biosensors

In addition to AI, biosensors will also be part of future CR programmes. Biosensors have many possible applications in cardiac healthcare. They can provide real-time monitoring and point of care diagnostic [47]. The combination with innovations like cardiac big data repositories, Internet of things-based applications and AI may help to develop new predictive models, create the ideal tailored programme and eventually act as a virtual assistant [47].

The ideal biosensor must be very specific, related to the specific health issues of the individual patient, and it should be able to transmit biomedical data wirelessly to the designated healthcare partner [48]. If these criteria are met, biosensors may be an ideal addition to every teleCR programme. With the use of applications based on the Internet of things incorporating biosensors for cardiac care as virtual assistants, patients can be monitored effectively and continuously. In this way, biosensors embedded with the machine-learning approach will facilitate the purpose of remote care and personalized medicine for effective diagnostics, rehabilitation, and follow-up [47].

References

1. Fletcher GF, Balady GJ, Amsterdam EA, et al. Exercise standards for testing and training: a statement for healthcare professionals from the American Heart Association. *Circulation* 2001; 104: 1694–1740.

2. Frederix I, Solmi F, Piepoli MF, et al. Cardiac telerehabilitation: a novel cost-efficient care delivery strategy that can induce long-term health benefits. *Eur J Prev Cardiol* 2017; 24: 1708–17.

3. Thorup C, Hansen J, Grønkjær M, et al. Cardiac patients' walking activity determined by a step counter in cardiac telerehabilitation: data from the intervention arm of a randomized controlled trial. *J Med Internet Res* 2016; 18: e69.

4. Osborn CY, van Ginkel JR, Marrero DG, et al. One Drop mobile on iPhone and Apple Watch: an evaluation of HbA1c improvement associated with tracking self-care. *JMIR Mhealth Uhealth* 2017; 5: e179.

5. Appelboom G, Camacho E, Abraham M, et al. Smart wearable body sensors for patient self-assessment and monitoring. *Arch Public Health* 2014; 72: 1–9.

6. Krittanawong Z, Zhang H, Wang Z, et al. Artificial intelligence in precision cardiovascular medicine. *J Am Coll Cardiol* 2017; 69: 2657–64.

7. Pevnick J, Birkeland K, Zimmer R, et al. Wearable technology for cardiology: an update and framework for the future. *Trends Cardiovasc Med* 2018; 28: 144–50.

8. Jimison H, Gorman P, Woods S, et al. *Barriers and Drivers of Health Information Technology Use for the Elderly, Chronically Ill, and Underserved*. Rockville, MD: Agency for Healthcare Research and Quality, 2008.

9. Mechanic OJ, Kimball AB. *Telehealth Systems*. Treasure Island, FL: StatPearls Publishing. Available from: https://www.ncbi.nlm.nih.gov/books/NBK459384/

10. Fletcher GF, Balady GJ, Amsterdam EA, et al. Exercise standards for testing and training: a statement for healthcare professionals from the American Heart Association. *Circulation* 2001; 104: 1694–1740.

11. Deering MJ. *Patient-Generated Health Data and Health IT. ONC Issue Brief*. Washington DC: Office of the National Coordinator for Health Information Technology, 20 December 2013.

12. Wang R, Blackburn G, Desai M, et al. Accuracy of wrist-worn heart rate monitors. *JAMA Cardiol* 2017; 2: 104.

13. Morgans CM, Rees JR. The action of perhexiline maleate in patients with angina. *Am Heart J* 1973; 86: 329–33.

14. Berlin JE, Storti KL, Brach JS. Using activity monitors to measure physical activity in free-living conditions. *Phys Ther* 2006; 86: 1137–45

15. Bravata DM, Smith-Spangler C, Sundaram V, et al. Using pedometers to increase physical activity and improve health: a systematic review. *JAMA* 2007; 298: 2296–304.

16. Evenson KR, Goto MM, Furberg RD. Systematic review of the validity and reliability of consumer-wearable activity trackers. *Int J Behav Nutr Phys Activity* 2015; 12: 159

17. Frederix I, Vanhees L, Dendale P. A review of telerehabilitation for cardiac patients. *J Telemed Telecare* 2015; 21: 45–53.

18. Richardson S, Mackinnon D. Left to their own devices? Privacy implications of wearable technology in Canadian workplaces. http://www.sscqueens.org/publications/left-to-their-own-devices.

19. Wagenaar RC, Sapir I, Zhang Y, et al. Continuous monitoring of functional activities using wearable, wireless gyroscope and accelerometer technology. *Conf Proc IEEE Eng Med Biol Soc* 2011; 2011: 4844–7.

20. Allen J. Photoplethysmography and its application in clinical physiological measurement. *Physiol Meas* 2007; 28: R1–39.

21. Kim SH, Ryoo DW, Bae C. Adaptive noise cancellation using accelerometers for the PPG signal from forehead. *Conf Proc IEEE Eng Med Biol Soc* 2007; 2007: 2564–7.

22. Reddy RK, Pooni R, Zaharieva DP, et al. Accuracy of wrist-worn activity monitors during common daily physical activities and types of structured exercise: evaluation study. *JMIR Mhealth Uhealth* 2018; 6: e10338

23. Degroote L, De Bourdeaudhuij I, Verloigne M, et al. The accuracy of smart devices for measuring physical activity in daily life: validation study. *JMIR Mhealth Uhealth* 2018; 6: e10972.

24. Krumholz HM, Merrill AR, Schone EM, et al. Patterns of hospital performance in acute myocardial infarction and heart failure 30-day mortality and readmission. *Circ Cardiovasc Qual Outcomes* 2009; 2: 407–13.

25. Adamson PB. Pathophysiology of the transition from chronic compensated and acute decompensated heart failure: new insights from continuous monitoring devices. *Curr Heart Fail Rep* 2009; 6:287–92

26. Amir O, Azzam ZS, Gaspar T, et al. Validation of remote dielectric sensing (ReDS) technology for quantification of lung fluid status: comparison to high resolution chest computed tomography in patients with and without acute heart failure. *Int J Cardiol* 2016; 221: 841–6.

27. Malfatto G, Villani A, Rosa FD, et al. Correlation between trans- and intra-thoracic impedance and conductance in patients with chronic heart failure. *J Cardiovasc Med* 2016; 17: 276–82.

28. Conraads VM, Tavazzi L, Santini M, et al. Sensitivity and positive predictive value of implantable intrathoracic impedance monitoring as a predictor of heart failure hospitalizations: the SENSE-HF trial. *Eur Heart J* 2011; 32: 2266–73.

29. Heist EK, Herre JM, Binkley PF, et al. Analysis of different device-based intrathoracic impedance vectors for detection of heart failure events (from the Detect Fluid Early from Intrathoracic Impedance Monitoring study). *Am J Cardiol* 2014; 114: 1249–56.

30. Beatty AL, Fukuoka Y, Whooley MA. Using mobile technology for CR: a review and framework for development and evaluation. *J Am Heart Assoc* 2013; 2: e000568.

31. Oinas-Kukkonen H, Harjumaa M. Towards deeper understanding of persuasion in software and information systems. *Proc 1st Int Conf on Advances in Computer–Human Interaction.* New York: IEEE, 2008, pp. 200–5.

32. Sankaran S, Dendale P, Coninx K. Evaluating the impact of the HeartHab app on motivation, physical activity, quality of life, and risk factors of coronary artery disease patients: multidisciplinary crossover study. *JMIR Mhealth Uhealth* 2019; 7: e10874. Available from: http://www.ncbi.nlm.nih.gov/pubmed/30946021

33. Stiggelbout AM, van der Weijden T, de Wit MPT, et al. Shared decision making: really putting patients at the centre of healthcare. *BMJ* 2012; 344: 28–31.

34. Kon AA. The shared decision-making continuum. *JAMA* 2010; 304: 903–4. Available from: https://doi.org/10.1001/jama.2010.1208

35. Patel MR, Dehmer GJ, Hirshfeld JW, et al. ACCF/SCAI/STS/AATS/AHA/ASNC 2009 Appropriateness Criteria for Coronary Revascularization: A Report by the American College of Cardiology Foundation Appropriateness Criteria Task Force, Society for Cardiovascular Angiography and Interventions, Society of Thoracic Surgeons, American Association for Thoracic Surgery, American Heart Association, and the American Society of Nuclear Cardiology Endorsed by the American Society of Echocardiography, the Heart Failure Society of America, and the

Society of Cardiovascular Computed Tomography. . *J Am Coll Cardiol* 2009; 53: 530–53. Available from: http://www.sciencedirect.com/science/article/pii/S0735109708033457

36. Allen LA, Stevenson LW, Grady KL, et al. Decision making in advanced heart failure: a scientific statement from the American Heart Association. *Circulation* 2012; 125: 1928–52.

37. Ottawa Hospital Research Institute. Alphabetical list of decision aids by health topic 2019. Available from: https://decisionaid.ohri.ca/AZlist.html

38. Joseph-Williams N, Elwyn G, Edwards A. Knowledge is not power for patients: a systematic review and thematic synthesis of patient-reported barriers and facilitators to shared decision making. *Patient Educ Couns* 2014; 94: 291–309. Available from: http://dx.doi.org/10.1016/j.pec.2013.10.031

39. Légaré F, Ratté S, Gravel K et al. Barriers and facilitators to implementing shared decision-making in clinical practice: update of a systematic review of health professionals' perceptions. *Patient Educ Couns* 2008; 73: 526–35.

40. Hess EP, Coylewright M, Frosch DL, et al. Implementation of shared decision making in cardiovascular care past, present, and future. *Circ Cardiovasc Qual Outcomes* 2014; 7: 797–803.

41. Allen LA, Matlock DD, Shetterly SM, et al. Use of risk models to predict death in the next year among individual ambulatory patients with heart failure. *JAMA Cardiol* 2017; 2: 435–41.

42. Shah RU, Rumsfeld JS. Big data in cardiology. *Eur Heart J* 2017; 38: 1865–7.

43. Krittanawong C, Zhang H, Wang Z, et al. Artificial intelligence in precision cardiovascular medicine. *J Am Coll Cardiol* 2017; 69: 2657–64.

44. *Oxford Dictionary of English* (3rd edn). Oxford: Oxford University Press, 2010.

45. Tajik AJ. Machine learning for echocardiographic imaging: embarking on another incredible journey. *J Am Coll Cardiol* 2016; 68: 2296–8.

46. Johnson KW, Torres Soto J, Glicksberg BS, et al. Artificial intelligence in cardiology. *J Am Coll Cardiol* 2018; 71: 2668–79.

47. Vashistha R, Dangi AK, Kumar A, et al. Futuristic biosensors for cardiac health care: an artificial intelligence approach. *3 Biotech* 2018; 8: 358.

48. Thévenot DR, Toth K, Durst RA, Wilson GS. Electrochemical biosensors: recommended definitions and classification 1. *Biosens Bioelectron* 2001; 16: 121–31.

Further reading

Piotrowicz E, Pencina MJ, Opolski G, et al. Effects of a 9-week hybrid comprehensive telerehabilitation program on long-term outcomes in patients with heart failure: The Telerehabilitation in Heart Failure Patients (TELEREH-HF) randomized clinical trial. *JAMA Cardiol* 2020; 5: 300–8.

Su J, Doris Y, Torralba Paguio J. Effect of eHealth cardiac rehabilitation on health outcomes of coronary heart disease patients: a systematic review and meta-analysis. *J Adv Nurs* 2020; 76:754–72.

Chapter 20

eHealth in cardiac rehabilitation

Ines Frederix and Paul Dendale

Summary

TeleCR is an innovative and (cost-)effective preventive care delivery strategy that can overcome the challenges associated with traditional centre-based cardiac rehabilitation (CR). This chapter describes how it can be implemented in daily practice. From an organizational point of view, it implies a shift in traditional and operational workflows and reorganization of the (non-)human resources for care delivery. The establishment of a well-coordinated tele-team, the definition of clear goals, profound progress monitoring and follow-up, and the creation of an environment that promotes sustained delivery of teleCR are paramount. Tackling the current legal and technological challenges is another prerequisite for successful implementation.

Introduction

Traditional centre-based CR programmes for patients suffering from coronary artery disease and/or heart failure are well established and evidence based [1–4]. As an addition to acute revascularization and optimal pharmacological treatment, multicomponent CR reduces mortality further [5]. Unfortunately, in clinical practice, patient uptake and adherence to centre-based CR remains suboptimal [6]. Cardiac patients are often unable and/or unwilling to attend these programmes because of transport problems, lack of time, and/or scheduling conflicts associated with their vocational reintegration. Community-based CR solves the transport problem, but often not the scheduling problem. eHealth-based care has been identified as a promising way of countering these challenges [7]. eHealth can be defined as 'the use of emerging information and communication technology to improve or enable health and healthcare delivery' [8]. It is used as a general term, encompassing eLearning, remote monitoring (i.e. tele-monitoring), structured telephone support, mHealth apps, and teleCR which is the focus of this chapter. TeleCR means rehabilitation from a distance. It combines remote monitoring of self-measured patient data (i.e. motion sensor data, blood pressure data, etc.), tele-coaching (i.e. coaching from a distance by email/SMS/telephone), eLearning, and social interaction [9]. Previous scientific research suggests that it can be an effective and cost-efficient additional treatment option for those patients who are not able to attend centre-based programmes and for long-term care provision [10–12]. The purpose of this chapter is to provide a framework and practical guide on how to implement teleCR in daily clinical practice.

How to implement cardiac tele-rehabilitation: organizational aspects

The implementation of cardiac teleCR implies several organizational issues, the most important of which are discussed in this section.

Change in traditional and operational workflows

The implementation of teleCR in clinical practice comes with changing roles and responsibilities for both patients and healthcare staff. In teleCR, a more patient-centric model of care applies. The cardiac patient adopts a more active role and becomes responsible for data registration and transmission to the central teleCR unit, where incoming data will be reviewed and feedback provided. This illustrates the importance of upfront identification of patient-related barriers for the use of eHealth applications [13–15]. Patient education about the teleCR programme should address their eHealth literacy skills and inform them about care quality assurance. Individual counselling may be needed to support and screen the patient, and to motivate them in case of hesitancy. From a healthcare provider perspective, tele-medical care programmes imply less in-person time to build and maintain the patient–caregiver relationship. Tele-paramedical personnel will become responsible for review of incoming data (i.e. can be both synchronous and asynchronous). If the data received deviates from what is expected, it will be necessary to inform the supervising CR specialist/cardiologist. Upfront clear accountability and liability rules/agreements should be defined. In addition, the responsibilities of other relevant staff members (e.g. supporting IT personnel) should be clarified. Standard operating procedures (SOPs) with a clear description of the teleCR workflow are mandatory.

Change in (non-)human resources necessary for care delivery

Implementation of teleCR will imply a shift in monetary resources. Currently, eHealth-based care delivery is only reimbursed in a few countries. Lack of reimbursement has been identified as one of the major barriers to the adoption of tele-medical care [16]. However, the National Health Fund in Poland finances some eHealth care programmes including hybrid teleCR, and in the Netherlands eHealth care has been reimbursed since January 2019. Early involvement of relevant financial institutions on a national level is essential. Several alternative business models should be explored. Pay for service in which the patient is charged directly for costs related to tele-medical care is an option. Patient clubs and private health insurance companies should be asked for their support if care remuneration remains absent.

How to implement cardiac tele-rehabilitation: practical aspects

From a practical point of view, several consecutive steps should be considered and addressed in order to ascertain successful implementation of cardiac teleCR in clinical practice [17].

Establishing an appropriate tele-team

A major change in healthcare delivery (of which teleCR is an example) needs a strong sponsoring committee together with a powerful guiding coalition, with the right composition, level of trust, and a shared objective of improving care quality. For example, the project could be sponsored by a tele-medical care sponsoring committee, composed of the chief of the cardiology division, the director of the CR centre, the chief cardiology nurse, and the hospital's medical director. Their task will be to communicate the need for teleCR and to mobilize commitment of team members. Team members can include appropriately trained and 'tele-certified' cardiac tele-nurses, tele-physiotherapists, tele-cardiologists, and/or teleCR specialists. They will monitor and supervise the cardiac patients remotely, supported by IT personnel who will ensure efficient functioning of both the tele-software and the tele-hardware.

Creating a vision and clarifying a goal

Defining a clear vision, driving the initiative fo change, and establishing a clear goal will help to inspire and motivate relevant stakeholders involved in the change in care delivery. The vision of improving quality of care by addressing more eligible CR patients can serve as an example. SMART (**S**pecific, **M**easurable, **A**chievable, **R**ealistic, **T**imed) rehabilitation goals are preferably used in order to increase the probability of goal attainment and to facilitate progress monitoring [18]. Improving the percentage of patients with optimal secondary prevention programme adherence by $x\%$, y months after the implementation of the cardiac teleCR programme is one example of a SMART goal.

Progress monitoring and follow-up

Monitoring the progress of the implementation process and adapting it if ncessary is one of the cornerstones of successful implementation. Repetitive Plan–Do–Study–Act (PDSA) cycling is a useful instrument for doing this [19]: **plan** the implementation process well in advance; **do** all the necessary things during the implementation process; **study** and monitor whether the implementation was successful; **act** accordingly (adopt/adapt/abandon the intervention). To monitor progress, consider both outcome and process metrics and the qualitative feedback from all stakeholders involved. The primary SMART goal can serve as the outcome metric as it reflects whether or not the implementation of the teleCR programme improved the quality of care. Process metrics are used to investigate whether the patients (and healthcare staff involved) actually adhered to the tele-programme (e.g. number of times daily data is uploaded). Qualitative feedback from all stakeholders involved will aid in deciding whether and how to change the current tele-programme to the next version, thereby increasing feasibility, acceptance and programme adoption.

Addressing obstacles blocking the implementation process

Upfront identification and handling of obstacles blocking the implementation process is paramount. Patient and caregiver resistance to change, resource constraints, and concerns related to whether or not the tele-medical care technology is fail-safe are some examples of possible obstacles. Understanding the reasons for resistance by active listening and open dialogue, and focusing corrective measures on the identified causes of resistance is a first step. On-site staff meetings can be used to provide resistant tele-personnel with objective outcome/process metric data from before, during, and after the teleCR implementation process.

Create an environment that promotes sustained delivery of tele-rehabilitation

If the implementation of teleCR is successful, the next goal is long-term sustainability. Supportive leadership, structural care change, continuous progress monitoring, and project outcome communication can help in this regard. The sponsoring committee has an important role in championing the new tele-medical care delivery strategy. Adequate resource allocation for the continuation of the teleCR unit is paramount. Repetitively reporting the initially defined outcome/process metrics and qualitative feedback to the sponsoring committee, the tele-personnel, other personnel in the hospital, and patients is another measure for keeping everybody informed about what has been accomplished.

How to cope with legal frameworks and changing technologies

When applying and implementing eHealth-based care in practice in Europe, a number of rules and legislation need to be taken into account. Directive 2016/679 (General Data Protection Regulation) with regard to the processing and free movement of personal sensitive data [20], the ePrivacy Directive (2002/58/EC) describing the applicable data protection principles [21], and Directive 2007/47/EC defining software for medical purposes as a medical device [22] are relevant to the application of teleCR in practice.

Innovations in information and communication technologies have enabled the establishment of eHealth care delivery. Numerous eHealth and mobile health applications are available, and technology is evolving very rapidly. However, implementing an eHealth programme (e.g. teleCR) in practice implies an organizational and workflow redesign, rather than just the introduction of the technological solution. In this sense, efforts should be focused on the operational organization around the teleCR programme, rather than on the changing technology.

Conclusion

TeleCR has been introduced recently as a result of innovations in telecommunication technologies. It encourages cardiac patients to take a more active role in their care programme under the remote supervision of relevant healthcare staff and can be applied as an additional care strategy to address those patients not able/willing to adhere to classical centre-based CR programmes. This chapter summarized the organizational and practical aspects that need to be taken into account when implementing cardiac tele-rehabilitation in practice, aiming to provide a clear guide on how to start the implementation process.

References

1. Ibanez B, James S, Agewall S, et al. 2017 ESC Guidelines for the management of acute myocardial infarction in patients presenting with ST-segment elevation: The Task Force for the management of acute myocardial infarction in patients presenting with ST-segment elevation of the European Society of Cardiology (ESC). *Eur Heart J* 2018; 39: 119–77.

2. Roffi M, Patrono C, Collet JP, et al. 2015 ESC Guidelines for the management of acute coronary syndromes in patients presenting without persistent ST-segment elevation. *Eur Heart J* 2016; 37: 267–315.

3. Montalescot G, Sechtem U, Achenbach S, et al. 2013 ESC guidelines on the management of stable coronary artery disease. *Eur Heart J* 2013; 34: 2949–3003.

4. Ponikowski P, Voors AA, Anker SD, et al. 2016 ESC Guidelines for the diagnosis and treatment of acute and chronic heart failure. *Eur Heart J* 2016; 37: 2129–200.

5. Rauch B, Davos CH, Doherty P, et al. The prognostic effect of cardiac rehabilitation in the era of acute revascularisation and statin therapy: a systematic review and meta-analysis of randomized and non-randomized studies—The Cardiac Rehabilitation Outcome Study (CROS). *Eur J Prev Cardiol* 2016; 23: 1914–39.

6. Kotseva K, Wood D, De Bacquer D, et al. EUROASPIRE IV: A European Society of Cardiology survey on the lifestyle, risk factor and therapeutic management of coronary patients from 24 European countries. *Eur J Prev Cardiol* 2016; 23: 636–48.

7. Piepoli MF, Corrà U, Dendale P, et al. Challenges in secondary prevention after acute myocardial infarction: a call for action. *Eur J Prev Cardiol* 2016; 23:1994–2006.

8. Pagliari C, Sloan D, Gregor P, et al. What is eHealth: a scoping exercise to map the field. *J Med Internet Res* 2005; 7: e9.

9. Frederix I, Vanhees L, Dendale P, et al. A review of telerehabilitation for cardiac patients. *J Telemed Telecare* 2015; 21: 45–53.

10. Kraal JJ, van den Akker-van Marle ME, Abu-Hanna A, et al. Clinical and cost-effectiveness of home-based cardiac rehabilitation compared to conventional, centre-based cardiac rehabilitation: Results of the FIT@Home study. *Eur J Prev Cardiol* 2017; 24: 1260–73.

11. Frederix I, Solmi F, Piepoli MF, et al. Cardiac telerehabilitation: a novel cost-efficient care delivery strategy that can induce long-term health benefits. *Eur J Prev Cardiol* 2017; 24: 1708–17.

12. Piotrowicz E, Baranowski R, Bilinska M, et al. A new model of home-based telemonitored cardiac rehabilitation in patients with heart failure: effectiveness, quality of life, and adherence. *Eur J Heart Fail* 2010; 12: 164–71.

13. Richtering SS, Hyun K, Neubeck L, et al. e-Health literacy: predictors in a population with moderate-to-high cardiovascular risk. *JMIR Hum Factors* 2017; 4: e4.

14. Ware P, Bartlett SJ, Paré G, et al. Using e-Health technologies: interests, preferences, and concerns of older adults. *Interact J Med Res* 2017; 6: e3.

15. O' Connor S, Hanlon P, O'Donnell CA, et al. Understanding factors affecting patient and public engagement and recruitment to digital health interventions: a systematic review of qualitative studies. *BMC Med Inform Decis Mak* 2016; 16: 120.

16. World Health Organization. *Atlas of e-Health Country Profiles: The Use of E-Health in Support of Universal Health Coverage: Based on the Findings of the Third Global Survey on e-Health 2015*. http://apps.who.int/iris/bitstream/10665/204523/1/9789241565219_eng.pdf?ua=1. Accessed 17 March 2018.

17. Kotter JP *Leading Change*. Boston, MA: Harvard Business School Press; 1996.

18. Bovend'Eerdt TJ, Botell RE, Wade DT. Writing SMART rehabilitation goals and achieving goal attainment scaling: a practical guide. *Clin Rehabil* 2009; 23: 352–61.

19. Lipshutz AK, Fee C, Schell H, et al. Strategies for success: a PDSA analysis of three QI initiatives in critical care. *Jt Comm J Qual Patient Saf* 2008; 34: 435–44.

20. Regulation (EU) 2016/679 of the European Parliament and of the Council. http://eur-lex.europa.eu/legal-content/EN/TXT/PDF/?uri=CELEX:32016R0679&from=EN. Accessed 17 March 2018.

21. Directive 2002/58/EC of the European Parliament and of the Council of 12 July 2002 concerning the processing of personal data and the protection of privacy in the electronic communications sector. http://eur-lex.europa.eu/legal-content/EN/TXT/?uri=CELEX%3A32004L0052. Accessed 20 March 2018.

22. Directive 2007/47/EC of the European Parliament and of the Council. http://eur-lex.europa.eu/LexUriServ/LexUriServ.do?uri=OJ:L:2007:247:0021:0055:en:PDF Accessed 17 March 2018.

Further reading

Frederix I, Caiani EG, Dendale P, et al. ESC e-Cardiology Working Group Position Paper: Overcoming challenges in digital health implementation in cardiovascular medicine. *Eur J Prev Cardiol* 2019; 26: 1166–77.

Chapter 21

The EXPERT tool: how to make exercise prescription easy

Dominique Hansen and Karin Coninx

Summary

Exercise training (ET) is a cornerstone of the multidisciplinary rehabilitation of patients with and at risk of cardiovascular disease (CVD). However, evidence indicates that clinicians experience difficulties in prescribing exercise for patients with different CVDs and risk factors (RFs). Different exercise intensities, duration, volume, frequency, and type will lead to different changes in CVD RFs. The Exercise Prescription in Everyday Practice & Rehabilitative Training (EXPERT) tool has been developed to overcome this limitation. It is a potential method for encouraging standardization of exercise prescription in CVD (risk) and enhancing the implementation of integrated exercise guidelines into clinical practice. The aim of this chapter is to guide clinicians on how to use the EXPERT tool to optimize their exercise prescription (skills).

Introduction

ET is a cornerstone of the multidisciplinary rehabilitation of CVD [1]. However, in order to maximize the impact of ET, exercise modalities should be selected carefully (e.g. intensity, frequency, volume, and type). Different exercise prescriptions will lead to different changes in exercise capacity, glycaemic control, blood pressure (BP), lipid profile, and adipose tissue mass [2].

When different CVDs and RFs are present within the same patient, clinicians experience difficulties on how to prescribe exercise to target these different CVDs and RFs simultaneously by means of ET. A recent European survey revealed a significant inter-clinician variance in exercise prescription for the same patients with different combinations of CVDs and RFs (Figure 21.1) [3]. This indicates that there is poor agreement between clinicians on how exercise should be prescribed to patients with CVD (risk) and that current CR exercise prescription is open to improvement.

As a result, if greater reductions in adipose tissue mass, blood lipids, and BP are desired, assistance in exercise prescription to patients with different CVDs and RFs is warranted [4–7].

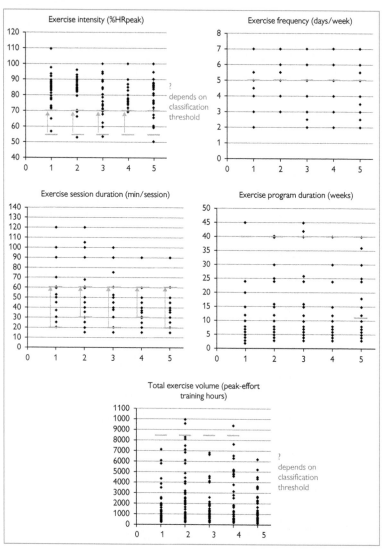

Figure 21.1 Inter-clinician variance in exercise prescription for the same five patient cases. Fifty-three CV rehabilitation clinicians from nine European countries were asked to prescribe exercise intensity (based on the percentage of peak heart rate (%HR$_{peak}$)), frequency, session duration, and programme duration to the same five patients. Exercise prescriptions were compared between clinicians, and these exercise prescriptions were compared with recommendations from the EXPERT tool (in grey). One point in the figure may reflect multiple clinicians, as similar exercise modality selections may have occurred between clinicians' lines.

Reproduced from Hansen D, Rovelo Ruiz G, Doherty P, et al. Do clinicians prescribe exercise similarly in patients with different cardiovascular diseases? Findings from the EAPC EXPERT working group survey. *Eur J Prev Cardiol* 2018; 25: 682–91 with permission from SAGE Publishing.

The EXPERT tool is a potential method for encouraging standardization of CR exercise prescription and enhances the implementation of integrated exercise guidelines into clinical practice. The aim of this chapter is to guide clinicians on how to use the EXPERT tool to optimize their exercise prescription (skills).

The EXPERT tool: features and functionalities

The EXPERT tool

The EXPERT tool is a training and decision support system, designed and built by computer scientists from the Expertise Centre of Digital Media, Hasselt University, in close collaboration with the EAPC EXPERT working group [8,9]. ET recommendations and safety precautions for ten CVDs, five CVD RFs, and three common chronic non-CV conditions are available in the EXPERT tool. It also takes the baseline exercise tolerance, common CV medications, and the occurrence of adverse events during exercise testing into account. The tool incorporates a training centre where clinicians can learn how to prescribe exercise to patients with CVD (risk). The exercise prescriptions of the EXPERT tool are based on clinical guidelines, evidence, and expert opinions collected by a working group of 33 CR specialists from 11 European countries. It automatically provides an exercise prescription depending on the characteristics of each patient case, thus integrating different exercise prescriptions for different CVDs and RFs within the same patient.

The EXPERT recommendation centre

The EXPERT tool has two working modes, the EXPERT recommendation centre and the EXPERT training centre, which function slightly differently. The EXPERT recommendation centre is the working mode used by a rehabilitation expert or clinician during a consultation or a supervised exercise session, or in the preparation for such an encounter. The EXPERT tool is a decision support tool, which allows the rehabilitation expert to enter the patient's personal data and different characteristics of their CV risk profile. Based on this input, the recommendation algorithm decides on an exercise prescription according to the European guidelines. The details of the exercise prescription (e.g. exercise intensity and frequency, session duration, programme duration, and the addition of strength training or other training modes) are presented to the rehabilitation expert at the EXPERT tool's user interface. In line with the concept of a decision-support tool, the rehabilitation expert can either work with the exercise recommendation proposed by the EXPERT tool or change the prescription's components to integrate their personal opinion and expertise. As well as showing the exercise recommendation that is based on European guidelines and expert opinions from members of the international EXPERT group, the EXPERT tool lists 'Safety precautions'. These are caveats for the rehabilitation experts—things to keep in mind during ET or to avoid because of specific patient characteristics. The fact that the EXPERT tool's recommendation is accompanied by safety precautions highlights the applicability of the prescription in day-to-day rehabilitation practice. This feature has been very well received in the CR community.

The design of the EXPERT tool's recommendation centre is optimized for easy and fast generation of an exercise prescription by a rehabilitation expert such as a cardiologist or physiotherapist. Figure 21.2 shows a typical screenshot of the EXPERT tool when the recommendation centre is activated. The upper part (light grey background) is a concise display of the patient data. The pen icon opens a pop-up window for editing the patient data. This is the first step when the EXPERT tool is used for a new patient, or when patient data have to be updated with the results of recent clinical tests (e.g. $VO_{2\,max}$ value is updated after a CPET to allow the EXPERT algorithm to recalculate the optimal exercise recommendation). Patient data is not generally updated frequently during an interactive session with the EXPERT tool when the rehabilitation expert is investigating the effect of the patient's RFs on the prescription.

The main area of the screen is allocated to the user interface elements which facilitate the process to formulate a specific personalized training prescription for the patient under consideration. At the same time, this approach stimulates the rehabilitation expert to interactively explore the contributing effects of different CVD RFs and diseases to the resulting EXPERT recommendation. When designing the overall concept of the EXPERT tool [8,9] it was decided to maximize exploitation of the possibilities of interactive exploration by the user, rather than merely visualizing an extensively branching tree showing conditions and decisions guiding the prescription rationale of a rehabilitation expert.

A number of horizontal panels denote the decisions that a rehabilitation expert will take to personalize the exercise prescription. Essentially, these are the factors that the EXPERT algorithm will consider to make a recommendation for the patient:

- starting by selecting the patient's primary index (e.g. coronary artery disease with or without percutaneous coronary intervention, coronary artery bypass grafting (CABG) or endoscopic atraumatic CABG surgery (endo-ACAB), heart failure (with preserved or lowered left-ventricular ejection fraction), cardiomyopathy, intermittent claudication, implantable cardioverter–defibrillator (ICD) or pacemaker, ventricular assist devices, heart transplantation, valve disease or surgery, congenital heart disease, pulmonary hypertension)

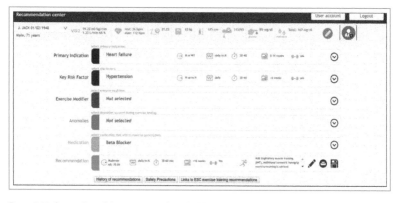

Figure 21.2 Screenshot of the main page of the EXPERT tool recommendation centre.
Courtesy of Dominique Hansen and Karin Coninx (EXPERT tool training and recommendation Hasselt University).

- adding information on key CVD RFs (e.g. types 1 and 2 diabetes mellitus, obesity, hypertension, hypercholesterolaemia/dyslipidaemia), exercise modifiers (sarcopenia, chronic pulmonary disease, or renal insufficiency/failure), abnormalities discovered during exercise (myocardial ischaemia, exercise-induced atrial fibrillation, and presence of ICD), and medication taken by the patient (beta-blockers, statins, exogenous insulin administration, or meglitinide/sulfonylurea).

Each panel has a brightly coloured zone to the left for easy visual discrimination, thus supporting fast interaction by the rehabilitation expert. By activating the arrow icon on the right-hand side, each panel functions as a drop-down box offering choices to the user (e.g. selecting a particular primary indication (Figure 21.3, or selecting HF as a primary indication).

Depending on the patient factor to be fixed, the drop-down boxes offer single selection or multiple selection interaction. If a factor is selected for this patient, the value is displayed on the left of the panel (Figure 21.2, the key RF is hypertension) and a prescription based on this contributing factor only is shown in the middle of the panel.

The key panel for the rehabilitation expert is the EXPERT recommendation panel, which is located below the five panels for the patient's RFs and contributing factors. The recommendation is visualized using icons and values for the separate components of the exercise prescription: exercise intensity, exercise frequency, session duration, programme duration, strength training, additional training (Figure. 21.2, horizontal 'Recommendation' panel at the bottom of the screen). It is important to emphasize that this recommendation is a combined result determined by the individual contributing factors, as outlined by the EAPC EXPERT group. It should be noted that any change in the contributing factors that is interactively made by the user instantaneously triggers a recalculation of the combined EXPERT recommendation. The easy interactive exploration of the contributing effects of individual patient factors and the proposed combined exercise recommendation (according to

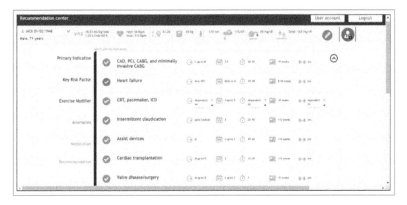

Figure 21.3 EXPERT recommendation centre: expanded dropdown box for selecting the primary indication.
Courtesy of Dominique Hansen and Karin Coninx (EXPERT tool training and recommendation Hasselt University).

European guidelines) are the major benefits of the EXPERT tool for individual and even experienced rehabilitation experts, particularly in complex cases,.

The recommendation can be manually edited (Figure 21.4) if the rehabilitation expert judges that the prescription proposed by the EXPERT tool should be overruled, in which case it is advisable to document the reasons for adapting the guideline-based recommendation for the patient under consideration. Once the desired prescription is achieved, it can be saved (using the disk icon) and exported/printed for inclusion in the patient's file (using the printer icon).

The lower part of the screen contains three buttons which activate history of recommendations, safety precautions, and links to ESC ET guidelines (Figure 21.2, grey buttons at the bottom). The history of recommendations provides a visualization of consecutive EXPERT recommendations that have been generated for this particular patient. In this way, an overview of the supervised (and possibly non-supervised) ET modalities is stored for future reference. The safety precautions that are generated next to the exercise prescription, ensure that the rehabilitation expert can instruct the patient to train with maximal safety. Links to ESC ET guidelines are references to published papers with ET guidelines. This demonstrates that the EXPERT tool is based on recognized guidelines. As well as incorporating these guidelines into day-to-day rehabilitation practice, the EXPERT tool contributes to standardizing the way exercise prescriptions are made.

The EXPERT tool is not only of value in the individual practice of a rehabilitation expert, it is also beneficial in a collaborative context. Indeed, rehabilitation centres and hospitals often involve (multidisciplinary) teams in patient treatment. Under the constraints of good ethical conduct and while respecting governmental and institutional regulations (e.g. Europe's GDPR in the context of privacy), a group of colleagues are able to share patient data. The EXPERT tool accommodates user group management and patient data sharing, including the saved exercise recommendations.

The version of the EXPERT tool described here functions as a stand-alone web-based application. Patient data input is generally done manually by the rehabilitation expert, but can also be entered by the support staff of the rehabilitation centre to

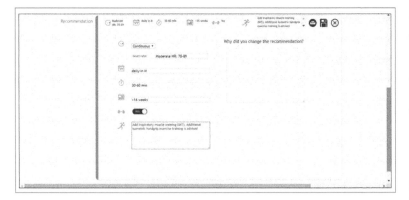

Figure 21.4 EXPERT recommendation centre: expanded panel for editing the recommendation.
Courtesy of Dominique Hansen and Karin Coninx (EXPERT tool training and recommendation Hasselt University).

allow the rehabilitation expert to focus on the clinical details, such as the patient's risk profile, and subsequently explore the recommendation generated by the EXPERT tool. In addition to this stand-alone version, proof-of-concept implementations have been realized in which the EXPERT tool is integrated into other medical information systems, for instance in the caregiver dashboard of a tele-rehabilitation system [10,11]. This integration or coupling with other medical information systems makes it possible to use patient data that are already stored rather than having to input these again. However, the easy user interface of the EXPERT tool speeds up data input, and the stand-alone tool has the advantage of being readily available (with an appropriate end-user licence) for individual rehabilitation experts or a group of colleagues in a rehabilitation setting.

The EXPERT training centre

The EXPERT training centre is the other working mode of the EXPERT tool. Exploring more than 60 fictional, but realistic, cases with different levels of complexity, a rehabilitation expert or trainee can become acquainted with do's and don'ts for exercise prescription for CV patients. They can check to what extent their exercise prescription behaviour is in line with the European guidelines incorporated in the EXPERT tool. Although the EXPERT training centre is a very valuable digital environment for cardiologists or physiotherapists in training, investigating fictional cases with increasing complexity is also valuable for experienced CR professionals.

The user interface of the EXPERT tool's training centre (Figure 21.5) is similar to the look and feel of the EXPERT recommendation centre, apart from the functionality of the recommendation panel. When working in the EXPERT training centre, the user selects a fictional case. The patient data corresponding to the case are displayed in the grey zone at the top of the EXPERT window, and the selected indications and contributing factors are displayed in the respective panels. However,

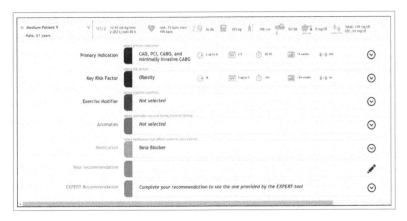

Figure 21.5 Screenshot of the main page of the EXPERT tool training centre.
Courtesy of Dominique Hansen and Karin Coninx (EXPERT tool training and recommendation Hasselt University).

before the EXPERT tool proposes a recommendation, the user has to enter their own prescription. The EXPERT tool's exercise prescription according to the guidelines is then shown in another recommendation panel below the user's prescription. In this way, the vertical alignment of the components of the exercise prescription of the user's prescription and the EXPERT recommendation can easily be compared. Safety precautions are also shown in the EXPERT training centre.

Conclusion

Although ET is effective in reducing mortality and morbidity in patients with CVD (risk), standardization in exercise prescription is warranted. In this chapter it is shown how the EXPERT tool can be used to help achieve this goal.

Acknowledgement

We would like to recognize the contribution of Gustavo Rovelo Ruiz, Hasselt University, to the technical realization and support for the clinical studies with the EXPERT tool. We are also grateful to Eva Geurts and Karel Robert for their role in the prototype stage. Finally, we would like to thank all the EXPERT working group members for their commitment and support in this project.

References

1. Piepoli MF, Hoes AW, Agewall S, et al. 2016 European Guidelines on cardiovascular disease prevention in clinical practice. *Eur J Prev Cardiol* 2016; 23: NP1–96.

2. Hansen D, Niebauer J, Cornelissen V, et al. Exercise prescription in patients with different combinations of cardiovascular disease risk factors: a consensus statement from the EXPERT Working Group. *Sports Med* 2018; 48: 1781–97.

3. Hansen D, Rovelo Ruiz G, Doherty P, et al. Do clinicians prescribe exercise similarly in patients with different cardiovascular diseases? Findings from the EAPC EXPERT working group survey. *Eur J Prev Cardiol* 2018; 25: 682–91.

4. Chen YC, Tsai JC, Liou YM, et al. Effectiveness of endurance exercise training in patients with coronary artery disease: a meta-analysis of randomised controlled trials. *Eur J Cardiovasc Nurs* 2017; 16: 397–408.

5. Pedersen LR, Olsen RH, Jürs A, et al. A randomized trial comparing the effect of weight loss and exercise training on insulin sensitivity and glucose metabolism in coronary artery disease. *Metabolism* 2015; 64: 1298–1307.

6. Gomadam PS, Douglas CJ, Sacrinty MT, et al. Degree and direction of change of body weight in cardiac rehabilitation and impact on exercise capacity and cardiac risk factors. *Am J Cardiol* 2016; 117: 580–4.

7. Ades PA, Savage PD, Toth MJ, et al. High-calorie-expenditure exercise: a new approach to cardiac rehabilitation for overweight coronary patients. *Circulation* 2009; 119: 2671–8.

8. Hansen D, Dendale P, Coninx K, et al. The European Association of Preventive Cardiology Exercise Prescription in Everyday Practice and Rehabilitative Training (EXPERT) tool: a digital training and decision support system for optimized exercise prescription in cardiovascular disease. Concept, definitions and construction methodology. *Eur J Prev Cardiol* 2017; 24: 1017–31.

9. Hansen D, Dendale P, Coninx K. The EAPC EXPERT tool. *Eur Heart J* 2017; 38: 2318–20.

10. Sankaran S, Luyten K, Hansen D, et al. Have you met your METs? Enhancing patient motivation to achieve physical activity targets in cardiac tele-rehabilitation. *Proc 32nd Int BCS Human Computer Interaction Conf (HCI 2018), Belfast 2018*. 10.14236/ewic/HCI2018.48.
11. Sankaran S, Dendale P, Coninx K. Evaluating the impact of the HeartHab app on motivation, physical activity, quality of life and risk factors of coronary artery disease patients: a multidisciplinary cross-over study. JMIR Mhealth Uhealth 2019; 7: e10874.

Further reading

Marcolino MAZ, Plentz RDM. Relevance and limitations of decision support systems for outpatient cardiac rehabilitation. *Biomed J Sci Tech Res* 2019; 12. doi: 10.26717/BJSTR.2019.12.002295.

Index

Tables, figures, and boxes are indicated by an italic *t*, *f*, and *b* following the page number.

The abbreviation CR is used for cardiac/cardiovascular rehabilitation.

187